STRONG AND LEAN

ALSO BY MARK LAUREN WITH JOSHUA CLARK

You Are Your Own Gym

Body by You

STRONG AND LEAN

9-MINUTE DAILY WORKOUTS TO BUILD YOUR BEST BODY: NO EQUIPMENT, ANYWHERE, ANYTIME

Mark Lauren and Joshua Clark

ST. MARTIN'S
ESSENTIALS
NEW YORK

The information in this book is not intended to replace the advice of the reader's own physician or other medical professional. You should consult a medical professional in matters relating to health, especially if you have existing medical conditions, and before starting, stopping, or changing the dose of any medication you are taking. Individual readers are solely responsible for their own health-care decisions. The author and the publisher do not accept responsibility for any adverse effects individuals may claim to experience, whether directly or indirectly, from the information contained in this book.

First published in the United States by St. Martin's Essentials, an imprint of St. Martin's Publishing Group

STRONG AND LEAN. Copyright © 2021 by Mark Lauren and Joshua Clark. All rights reserved. Printed in the United States of America. For information, address St. Martin's Publishing Group, 120 Broadway, New York, NY 10271.

www.stmartins.com

Library of Congress Cataloging-in-Publication Data

Names: Lauren, Mark, 1972- author. | Clark, Joshua, 1975– author.
Title: Strong and lean : 9-minute daily workouts to build your best
    body—no equipment, anywhere, anytime / Mark Lauren and Joshua Clark.
Description: First edition. | New York : St. Martin's Essentials, 2021. |
Identifiers: LCCN 2021016083 | ISBN 9781250787194 (trade paperback) | ISBN
    9781250787200 (ebook)
Subjects: LCSH: Physical fitness. | Exercise.
Classification: LCC GV481 .L38 2021 | DDC 613.7—dc23
LC record available at https://lccn.loc.gov/2021016083

Our books may be purchased in bulk for promotional, educational, or business use. Please contact your local bookseller or the Macmillan Corporate and Premium Sales Department at 1-800-221-7945, extension 5442, or by email at MacmillanSpecialMarkets@macmillan.com.

First Edition: 2021

10 9 8 7 6 5 4 3 2 1

For our agent Steve Ross.

We can't imagine a better guide on such an amazing worldwide journey.

CONTENTS

INTRODUCTION

You hold in your hands the most direct path to an athlete's body, one that takes only 0.3 percent of your time each week.

Here's a simple truth: You achieve your best body through training the movements most important to your survival. But other trainers and authors haven't even asked what those are.

So I'm going to share with you what it took me a lifetime to find—the formula to the most desirable physique. It's almost sad that it's so secret. But the fitness industry doesn't want you to know the simple solution to reaching your goals, so they can keep you addicted to their gyms, equipment, and other needlessly complex, moneymaking fads.

Strong and Lean has proven to build more muscle than weight lifting, burn more fat than cardio, and produce sexier and safer results than either of those. It will turn your body into the only fitness equipment you'll ever need again.

I was proud to write the first bestselling bodyweight fitness book, *You Are Your Own Gym: The Bible of Bodyweight Exercises.* It was also the first popular fitness book based on a military program, and the first I know of to chuck out monotonous, time-consuming, energy-draining and inefficient cardio. *You Are Your Own Gym* remains a timeless resource for everything from body composition to motivation to nutrition. With 125 possible exercises, it transforms any room into a total fitness center.

Strong and Lean is a different animal. While *You Are Your Own Gym* is the "Bible of Bodyweight Exercises," *Strong and Lean* streamlines my life's work into one program in a simple layout, removing the guesswork. And while *You Are Your Own Gym* allows you to isolate muscle groups, here I've carefully engineered new movements that each strengthen your entire body at once.

Strong and Lean applies Western cutting-edge sports science to the Eastern world's wisdom, and couples that with three decades of unparalleled experience, so you only have to put in nine minutes a day, a few days a week. Never before has there been such a short, low-impact program that comprehensively and methodically covers all the muscle groups, joint functions, and athletic skills you require to get and stay strong, lean, healthy, mobile, and injury-free.

BUILDING A BILLION BEAUTIFUL BODIES: MISSION IMPOSSIBLE?

Doing my exercises in *You Are Your Own Gym,* millions have now used the body they had to build the body they wanted. But what about a billion? What's stopping so many people from having their best body?

Two things:

Those who work out:

Everyone wants to get leaner and stronger. But their goals always seem just out of reach. Why? Because most trainers and authors don't understand what *strength* actually means, and therefore how it's achieved while building your leanest body.

Those who don't work out:

Sedentary lifestyles and poor nutrition have thrust us into a health crisis that's making millions miserable, often leading to their early deaths. Everyone knows the benefits of consistent, proper exercise; you get healthier, stronger, leaner, sleep better, live longer, have more energy and more desire. So what's stopping them from doing it?

We conducted a survey asking just that. We asked a thousand Americans from all fifty states who didn't work out: why not? The number one answer? You may have guessed it: They say they don't have *time.*

So as *You Are Your Own Gym* became a bestseller in over a dozen countries, I set out on a worldwide mission, one even I thought impossible:

Could I develop the ultimate program that takes the least amount of time *and* produces the results people need?

MY JOURNEY

Like a lot of people, I've tried a lot of things that didn't work. I spent a life driving myself to extremes, trying to find the formula to the best human body. By the time I was nine, I was doing six hundred sit-ups a day on my bedroom floor. In high school, I competed in bodybuilding competitions. By the age of twenty, I'd become another gym bunny, developing undesirable proportions, mistaking the size of my muscles for actual ability and strength. I realized it wouldn't be long before I also developed debilitating chronic injuries. I saw firsthand that most bodybuilders can't even walk straight. So I started doing CrossFit-type workouts for hours every week before CrossFit was cool. Then I'd take Sunday off and play a sport with some guys and gals who don't even work out, and guess what? They'd kick my ass![*] I couldn't believe it. All that work wasn't paying off. The incredible inefficiency of my exercise programs really pissed me off. But the worst was yet to come.

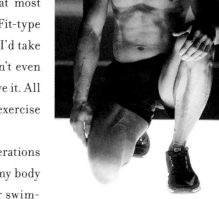

When I joined the air force, and eventually the Special Operations community, I prided myself on shutting out pain and taking my body past perceived limits. I still hold the U.S. military record for swimming underwater the longest (two minutes, twenty-three seconds), before blacking out underwater. Most of our Special Operations courses were designed to drive candidates into the floor. But only by realizing more is not better did I get better results. Because doing more than what's necessary only prolongs recovery and increases the risk of injury.

After serving on Silver Team at the 22nd Special Tactics Squadron at McChord AFB in Tacoma, Washington, I became the physical trainer of nearly a thousand elite Special Operations warriors—including SEALs, Rangers, Green Berets, Force Recon teams, and air force commandos—assigned to carry out the most dangerous missions. My men became my heroes. Some earned Silver Stars. They became the strongest and leanest people of our civilization. Because it wasn't their livelihoods but their *lives* (and ours) that depended on it.

---

[*] CrossFit, like most other programs out there, will cause some muscle adaptation, but it won't make you a better athlete in other sports, because the postural strategies for exercises like overhead squats, bench pressing, or timed pull-ups are not what you need to excel in real-life activities. So these programs created physical imbalances that deprived me of an athletic, capable body, which is always the best-proportioned, best-looking body.

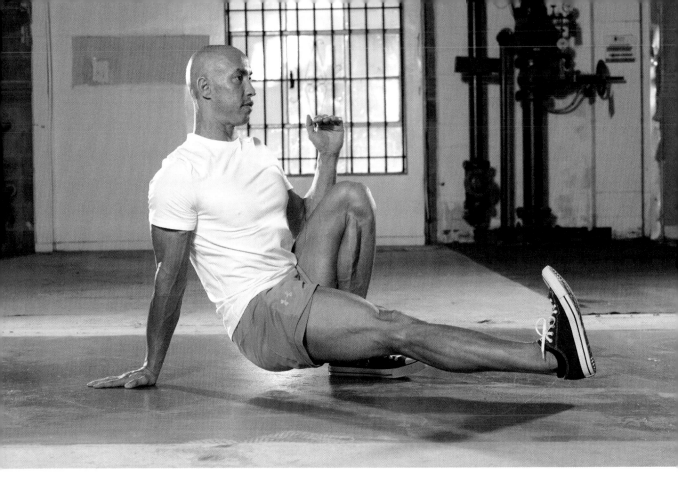

I developed a purely bodyweight program that evolved until my squadrons were using it not only in the field but even when equipment was available. One time, we actually gave away a few hundred thousand dollars' worth of exercise equipment, just to make room for more floor space. Because your arms were made to push and pull your bodyweight, not to grasp handles on machines or metal bars while you sit on a cushy bench. I mean, lying down on a soft surface is fine when you're sleeping. Sitting on a cushioned seat is fine if you're driving or looking at your computer or TV. But we realized we sure as hell shouldn't be doing that if we're doing real exercise.

You Are Your Own Gym brought my system to civilians—125 exercises for every single body part that transformed your living room, bedroom, office, garage, yard, you name it, into a total-body fitness center, using no equipment but the most efficient fitness device ever created: your own body.

My journey from military trainer to international bestselling author was a dream come true. It's been awesome getting real-time feedback from hundreds of thousands of social media subscribers. I've had the opportunity to train thousands of people, certify hundreds of trainers, and train the trainers of trainers. I got a ringside seat beside the men and women at the forefront of elite training and sports science. But more than all the science I studied and the research I conducted, experience inspired me most: from Dubai to Laos, from Afghanistan to Portland, from doing Dive Bomber Push-Ups in Moscow's Red Square in the snow and dark of the Russian winter to teaching coaches at the Chinese Olympic Training Center in Beijing.

I amassed all the pieces to the giant fitness puzzle. But it remained just that: in pieces. One big, needlessly complicated mess. There was a lot of good info out there from a lot of high-level strength and conditioning coaches I worked with. But incredibly, no one seemed able to distill the essence of what it truly takes to become strong and lean into something simple yet comprehensive that can be easily understood and applied.

I needed to go back to how I planned missions in the military:

Start with the objective, then work backward to find the most efficient strategy to achieve it.

OBJECTIVE: TO BUILD YOUR BEST BODY

STEP 1

SO WHAT EXACTLY DOES THE BEST BODY LOOK LIKE?

We find the most *capable* body the most *beautiful*. Because we've evolved to desire most those who not only survive but protect and take care of us. Therefore, the most functional program produces the best body. The reason weight lifting rarely produces the sexiest bods is that it's rarely useful outside the gym, where performance actually matters. But when you gain muscle through highly functional training, your body displays your self-mastery, which leads to mastery of your environment, and that is exactly what we need to survive and reproduce.

If someone built a bridge out of balloons, you'd probably notice something's not right with it before you drove over it. Building your best body is indeed like building a bridge. The long-term integrity and real strength needed to safely withstand day-to-day stress come

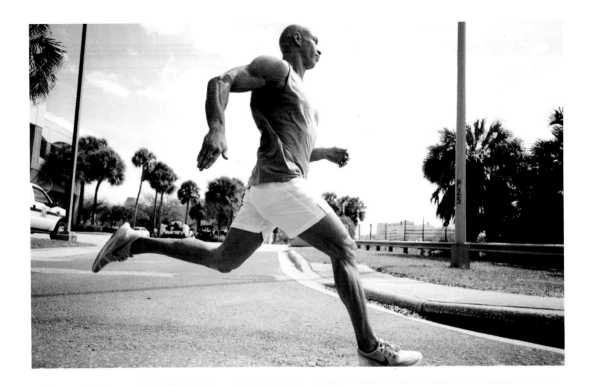

from the ideal alignment of your parts. Only by understanding and applying the fundamentals to real athletic ability and strength do we build a structure capable of supporting ourselves, and not only surviving but excelling at life and looks. Conversely, mistaking bigger muscles for useful athletic ability is like spending a ton of time building a bridge for looks alone. But then as soon as someone walks on it, it collapses beneath them. Literally. I dare you to take the biggest guy from any gym on a long walk. They probably aren't going to make it.

Even if you're into huge, bulky, disproportionate muscles and bad posture, you'd better be ready to do steroids as well. Many people would be shocked to know just how commonly, even casually, steroids are used in the weight lifting world. It's a sad fact that most of the humongous dudes you see in gyms are on them. But after a brief period in the '80s and '90s when roid-injected action heroes made the big bucks on the big screen, lean is sexy again. Just as lean was sexy for all one hundred thousand years of human history before steroids and "bodybuilding."

Society once again most desires the symmetry and proportions of actual athletes. As fashion and film and consistent polling show, everyone wants (and wants to be with) the athlete's bod—strong, lean, agile, and *useful* outside the gym, in sports and real life.

So which athletes would you say have the best physiques?

I'd argue NFL running backs, receivers, rugby players, ballerinas, and Olympic sprinters.

What do they all have in common?

They're really freaking good at getting from point A to point B.

So what skills do you need for that?

`STEP 2`

WHAT SKILLS DO YOU NEED TO GET THE BEST BODY?

True strength and ability can be summarized in a single word:

Locomotion the skill of moving from one place to another

synonyms: moving · traveling · mobility · progress · headway · action

Locomotion is one of the first things we learn as babies and one of the first we lose when we grow old (or lift too many weights). It's what you do every time you take a step, walk, run, sprint, climb, strike, throw, punch, kick, bowl, swing a club, or get off the ground.

Locomotion is the ultimate function. Because it makes you good at more things than any other skill. It is the single skill we use most. It is the most necessary skill to our survival and well-being, hence it produces the most desirable bodies. More than anything else in existence, locomotion impacts our life and looks.

`STEP 3`

SO HOW DO YOU IMPROVE LOCOMOTION?

How do we develop great-looking bodies by improving the skill we've evolved to find sexiest?

By understanding how we absorb, transfer, and generate force to get from place to place, without wasted effort.

I spent two decades either studying locomotion firsthand (with athletes and their trainers), observing it (particularly how differently people move in different cultures), or applying it to survive (as a Special Operations trainer, a warrior, and as a pro fighter). At every step of the way, I asked, to excel, *What exact body parts must we move? And how must we move them?*

I realized that when a joint is in the middle (neutrally aligned), all movement options are instantly available, and thus you can develop the most strength. Most strength-training programs don't consider this, and you therefore lose a lot of joint functions. Heavy squatters, for example, often lose internal hip rotation. Too much bench pressing gets you stuck in shoulder protraction with a forward head posture. Your body adapts to hard repetitive movements by increasing the tension of the muscles in use, which gets your joints stuck in extreme ranges of motion and pulls you out of ideal alignment for everything else. That's also true for hard bodyweight exercises if not balanced properly.

But I didn't want to add to the sports science Tower of Babel. I sought to reduce the locomotion to its simplest nature. I formulated the fundamental strategy of how humans can move better.

I first unveiled my strategy in Zurich, Switzerland, in 2018: The strongest and leanest bodies are best achieved through moving your hips and shoulders around a neutrally aligned spine, in a coordinated manner, that results in side-to-side weight shifting.

I'm going to teach you to get good at this:

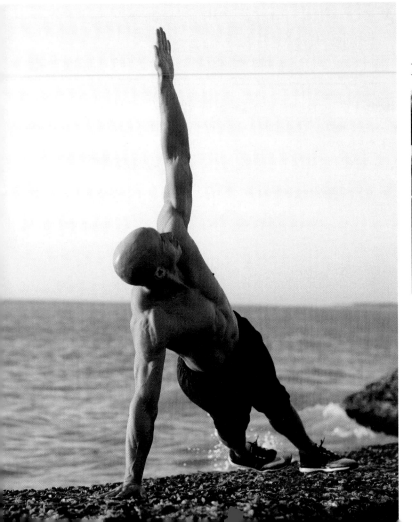

Not this:

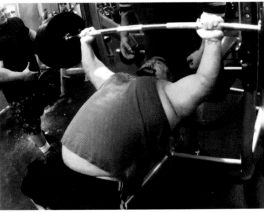

THEN HOW DO WE IMPROVE LOCOMOTION *QUICKEST*?

By simplifying. And that's the secret to this program.

WHY THEY LIE

In an already overly busy and complicated world, I've watched fitness fads getting more complex, while our society is getting in worse shape. And a lot of modern exercise fads are just too damn hard. Why? Because they're trying to overcome their lack of knowledge of what's really needed with sheer intensity and volume (whether that's long workout times or three-hundred-page books). It's like when you're in a chopper, taking incoming enemy fire, but you can't see where the enemy is hiding in the terrain below, so you just fire your .50-caliber machine gun all over the place: "Spray and pray, baby!"

"Spray and pray"—*rat-a-tat-tat-tat*—is a horribly inefficient approach to fitness. People are giving away *so* much of their money, time, and energy to get fit, without reaching their goals. And I see a fitness industry that frankly doesn't give a damn.

The industry makes its money by keeping us focused on isolating muscles and counting calories. Even those programs that use many muscles at once are mostly useless or counterproductive to real-life performance. It's crucial to them that we never reach our goals or change our way of thinking, because then we'd stop giving them our time and money.

Unlike other fitness "experts," I wanted *not* to create complex ways to make people suffer but instead to hone the absolute easiest and simplest solution to true, lasting fitness while looking awesome as fast as humanly possible, by accurately targeting our needs to get more for less.

YOU ONLY GET GOOD AT WHAT YOU DO

It was my boxing training in Thailand that drove this lesson home. I would see teenage Thai boxers manhandle much bigger and "stronger" men. It wasn't even close! For instance, while one sixteen-year-old was getting ready for a big fight, his trainer had him take turns on me and three other foreigners. In Thai boxing, you're allowed to do some limited upright wrestling and throwing in what's called the "clinch." Each time this kid threw one of us to the floor, the next foreigner would jump in the ring. No rest for the winner. But we never got him to the floor once. While your average person gasses out in thirty seconds of boxing, this kid stayed in the center of that ring for forty-five minutes as we rotated in and out, huffing and puffing. We all outweighed him by at least thirty pounds. And the crazy part is that he couldn't bench his own bodyweight!

These Thai boxers could stand directly in front of me and land a shin on my neck. Yet when it came to static stretching—which only the foreigners did—they could barely touch their own toes! It blew my mind.

I realized I wouldn't get good at Thai boxing by doing curls and hitting the StairMaster. Instead, I became a professional Thai boxing champion by Thai boxing. It seems obvious, right? But no, our society equates strength in the gym with performance in real life and real sports (actual ability that we've evolved to find sexy), but it's just marketing hype and nonsense.

The most effective way to train for something is by doing the actual thing you're training for.[*]

STEP 5

HOW DO YOU BECOME A CHAMPION AT LIFE?

So how do you become good at not just Thai boxing or bench pressing or running but the ability to move through life like an athlete?

As a young Special Ops guy, it was my job to be ready for all types of missions and environments at a moment's notice. On any given training cycle, we might jump out of the back of a plane at twelve thousand feet, wearing 130 pounds of gear and night vision goggles, skydiving after Harley-Davidson dirt bikes they'd just chucked out—strapped to pallets with parachutes attached—which we'd use the instant we hit the ground to practice rapid airfield seizures. A day later, we could be diving off the shores of Hawaii. And then summiting Mount Rainier the same week. We were supposed to be ready for everything.

But as I focused on one skill, the others would quickly detrain. If I ran a lot, my strength would decrease. If I focused on strength training, my running and swimming would suffer. If I tried to do everything at once, nothing would get to a very high level, because the types of adaptation opposed one another and time is limited.

The Special Operations community tries to overcome this problem by creating a lot of

---

[*] That's why using fitness machines makes you good at using fitness machines and not much else. In fact, there have been a few times I've mistakenly thought some of my clients were handicapped until I learned they were trainers who exclusively used fitness machines. Machines create learning disabilities because they limit your movement options and thereby impair your coordination. Contraptions don't train your body to function as a cohesive whole outside the gym, and so you develop ineffective motor patterns.

extra difficulty for new trainees, so that they are forced to adapt through coordinated effort, intelligent problem-solving, and, very often, sheer willpower. In other words, trainees are challenged with as much intentional inefficiency as possible to develop problem-solving skills that can be applied anywhere. This is effective, but attrition is high. There are few people able to deal with so much seemingly unnecessary stress that does not directly improve the operational tasks that really matter.

My first obvious lesson came immediately after graduating the Pararescue / Combat Control Indoctrination Course, one of the toughest selection courses in the military, when I strapped on a sixty-pound pack for the first time. The week before, I had broken the underwater record by swimming 133 meters subsurface on a single breath. By almost any measure, I was in superhuman condition, but I had never *rucked,* the military term for walking with a heavy pack. The lesson was instant and powerful. I could barely keep up with my peers whom I had easily outpaced in every single event during selection. All that training was for nothing when it came to getting from point A to point B with gear. Again, locomotion was the essential skill.

This environment ingrained in me a constant need to simplify and reduce, so that problems can be solved with minimal effort by focusing only on the essentials. And when I took command of the physical training, I worked hard to make training not complexer but smarter. These lessons later allowed me to cut through the complexity and nonsense of the fitness industry as well.

So if you only get good at what you do, then how is it possible to create an exercise program that effectively prepares you for just about everything? This is the functional training riddle that has gone unanswered for too long.

The answer: by isolating the precise, specific fundamentals that are needed for locomotion, and only focusing on those. This would mean with only a few minutes a day, you could indeed get better at everything.

But how do you simplify a billion dollars' worth of complex sports science down to those fundamentals?

WHEN I WAS LEAST EXPECTING IT

I was training in Indonesia, planning my upcoming bodyweight training courses in Germany, a requirement for their physical therapists, when the director of the Queen Rania Rehabilitation Center, a large and prestigious clinic at the Sport University of Cologne, reached out to me. A few months later in Germany, I took a lunch break to meet with her and her boss. Many had reached out from similar institutions. I always looked forward to helping them, and in turn learning from them and their athletes. But they had a very different idea.

They asked me to tour their center for children with cerebral palsy. I soon learned it was considered the leading clinic in the world for children with permanent movement disorders. Many had no locomotion at all. The children spent all day training with renowned therapists, day in and day out. The care and technology these kids received amazed me. We paused our tour of the facility to watch a young boy named Fabien suspended in a monstrous, complex, computerized, sci-fi-looking machine that made him walk, something he would never do on his own.

"But can he even get up off the ground?" I asked.

The director shook her head.

Then you might as well put this kid in a flying machine. No, I didn't say that out loud. But it was like having a machine force your hand to write calculus equations when you don't know what $1 + 1$ equals.

The next day, they let me spend an hour with nine-year-old Fabien. He took one look at me in my little black gym shorts and groaned, "Are we doing more leg presses today?"

Yes, they'd had a boy who had never walked doing leg presses. And he didn't look too happy about it. What struck me immediately was that I'd seen this same tendency in top athletes; many are notoriously lazy about strength and conditioning. They naturally understand what they need and what they don't, and they save their energy for the field, because actually doing the thing you're training for matters most. A lot of great athletes are great not because of their strength and conditioning programs but despite them.

I carried Fabien to a training mat and laid him on his side in a cradle position with his knees stacked and pulled up toward his chest. At first, he could barely lift his top knee off the bottom knee, which requires external hip rotation. But he was an extremely bright and motivated kid. We worked on this until he could open his legs quickly and actually resist me pushing down against his knee. After more isolated joint functions in lying positions, I got him rolling. We then worked movement by movement to get him from a front lying position to a crawling position. I showed him how to shift his weight to get his leg under him and build up into a full crawling position. After an hour, I watched Fabien get up off the floor by himself for the first time in his life.

I choked back tears, trying to remain professional. Fabien's own eyes filled not with tears but wonder.

And I realized I just might be looking at the solution to the great fitness riddle. Because here it was—all the scientific complexities of functional strength training simplified to their most fundamental essence. By stripping away everything that wasn't needed, I'd put into practice what I believed were the common denominators of locomotion. And watched a boy move in a way the world told him would never be possible.

STEP 6

THE SIMPLEST SOLUTION TO THE COMPLEX PROBLEM

Working with these kids was just too awesome. Their minds were sharp. Their wills strong. They knew what they dreamed of doing with their bodies but had never been shown how. So I flew back to Germany the next month, stayed longer at the clinic, and designed a program for them. I saw it time and again, these kids who had been unmotivated to do traditional strength training eagerly practiced the movements I showed them. Because they intuitively knew they needed them. The reward is instant, which drives the needed behavior. Their reactions to newly conquered positions were like an infant who rolls onto his belly for the first time and sees the world from a new viewpoint.

It was the ultimate irony: Children with cerebral palsy were validating my methods for attaining peak athletic performance as quickly and easily as possible.

But I wanted to put my methods to the test on the other extreme of the spectrum. So I went to work with the elderly in assisted-living facilities. While the children in Cologne had never before learned the fundamental athletic skills, these elderly had lost them, and so their lives were rapidly declining. When I got to one facility in Portland, they were playing with little pink dumbbells and doing water aerobics, "spraying and praying." Their trainers were simply trying to slow down the regression of their athletic skills with movements totally unrelated to their actual needs. Father Time is unstoppable, right?

By creating a progression out of the exact movements I believe you need to transition between lying and standing positions, I trained an eighty-four-year-old woman to get off the floor and walk without a cane for the first time in twenty years.

I realized that if I could teach these people to move in ways previously thought impossible, by applying the same methodology, I could turn the everyday person into an athlete. And I soon began doing so. Because the everyday person's learning curve is far less steep, and their potential far greater.

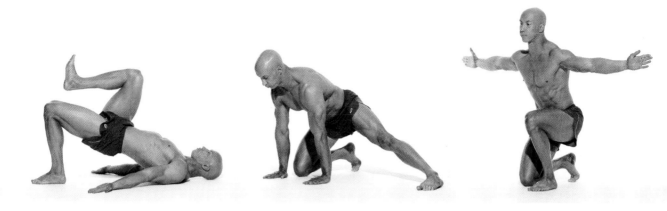

THE SECRET

I taught Fabien to get up off the ground by using the *exact* movements he needed each step of the way. I then drilled each movement he needed by making exercises out of them. Then I showed him how to put the simpler parts together into complexer movements like rolling, building up to crawling, then kneeling, and eventually getting off the ground.

This is how I learned to build the best bodies—by drilling only the movements that accurately duplicate what we need to move like athletes as efficiently as possible, and then stringing them together in the perfect progressions.

We combine letters of the alphabet to make words, and then words to make sentences. So, too, we must combine the isolated functions of our joints into whole-body movements. But it doesn't stop there. Just as sentences combine to form language, *Strong and Lean* then merges those whole-body exercises into dynamic, flowing movements that lean and strengthen your entire body most efficiently.

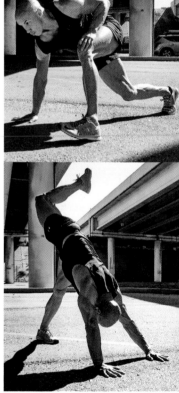

Conversely, bursting blood vessels on a bench press or exhausting yourself on a treadmill leaves you going nowhere, literally and figuratively. These isolated motions are like only being able to recite the alphabet, over and over and over.

Obviously, most of us don't yet face the same hurdles as the elderly. That's why the movements in this book's program are far complexer and more dynamic, and require and create more strength than the ones I implemented in rehabilitation centers. But we are applying the same fundamentals that will produce similarly dramatic results. And with you, the sky's the limit.

WHY STRENGTH TRAINING
AND NOT CARDIO

Again, look at evolution. Jogging, like weight lifting, poorly imitates actual athletic ability. Our prehistoric ancestors wanted a partner who could climb, sprint, track, hunt, strike, and throw a spear at things they could eat. That's whose children they wanted to have. No one gave a damn about "steady-state aerobics" or jogging. That's why most joggers don't have great bods.

The secret to reducing body fat is regaining your youthful metabolism by regaining your muscle. Muscle is the most metabolically expensive tissue we have; it takes between fifty and one hundred calories a day just to keep one pound of muscle alive, for both men and women. An extra five pounds of muscle can burn up to fifteen thousand calories in a month—that's the equivalent of two pounds of fat. Increased muscle mass lets you lose weight with less attention paid to calorie counting and food selection. Not only because of the muscle it builds but also the effect it has on the metabolism *following* the workouts—even while sleeping!

But if you plod along on a treadmill, you might go forty-five minutes before it says you burned 300 calories. Well, the average male burns 140 calories per hour at rest. The treadmill *actually* burned only 160 calories more than if you had been taking a nap. And aerobic exercise typically spurs your appetite enough to more than offset those few calories burned.

Whether running, cycling, or a step class, for the most part, it doesn't get easier because of muscular or cardiovascular endurance, but only because your body becomes more efficient at that particular movement. Again, you only get good at what you do. That's why cyclists will huff and puff if they jog for the first time in years. The body has no demand for extra muscle beyond what is needed to perform that relatively easy movement over and over. So your body adapts by actually burning muscle.

With consistent aerobic exercise, over time, you're more likely to *burn* five pounds of muscle. That means your body would burn 250 *fewer* calories a day. And as your body becomes more efficient at running, that 160 calories you burn on the treadmill will decrease to about 100.

So let's do the math. You burn 100 calories above your resting metabolic rate each day you do aerobic exercise. Then add the 250 calories you do not burn due to muscle loss caused by this exercise. After all your huffing and puffing, you are now 150 calories in the wrong direction!

Honestly, I'd rather sit in traffic for an hour than spend that time in the "fat-burning zone" on an elliptical. My program changes day to day, week to week. Play whatever music you want, and work out wherever makes you happiest.

PERFORMANCE = EFFICIENCY

For those seeking to lose fat, it's incredibly inefficient to exercise for the sake of burning calories. An hour on a treadmill can be undone by a slice of bread. So it's a lot more efficient just to eat a little less and build power and speed with my *STRONG & LEAN* program. Burn more fuel (calories), even while you sleep. And if you're worried about cardiovascular conditioning, my nine-minute program will build that, too.

Keep what gets results best and chuck the rest. Reducing training to only the most essential bodyweight movements nearly eliminates the cost in time and money while increasing the returns. Just like professional athletes do, you'll attain the most strength and the leanest body through the movements most vital to our survival.

SEXIER *AND SAFER*

Just as it's no coincidence the most functional exercises produce the most desirable bodies (evolution made it so), it's also no coincidence the most functional exercises are the safest. In a matter of weeks, many of my clients have eradicated knee, hip, shoulder, and neck pain.

Our bodies are essentially bunches of sticks (bones) stacked vertically. It's a marvel they stand up on their own! Think of your body as a long radio tower held up by cables going to the ground. If all the cables are perfectly proportioned and taut, the tower stands straight and strong. But if a single cable is unstable, not in tune with the others, the whole tower can topple. When this happens in your body, your brain sends out pain signals (in your knees, back, hips, neck, shoulders, etc.), and your posture starts going awry. The key is not developing crazier exercise machines and routines but developing a program that actually strengthens and integrates all these "cables."

Your body is like any other structure. Its ability to resist stress depends on the ideal alignment of its parts. Making this look simple took me years. Because, unlike a tower or building, which are static structures, your body's alignment is a fluid and constantly changing thing.

MOTIVATION?

I've never been big on trying to motivate people. As a gatekeeper to our Special Operations forces, my job was to make people quit, not to motivate them. Even when we tried to increase our graduate numbers by decreasing the number of pull-ups, push-ups, sit-ups, and running they had to do, our numbers didn't change. I've seen it time and again, both in the military and in the civilian world—whoever is going to make it, is going to make it. You're either going to take the nine minutes a day to become lean and strong, or you're not. Nothing I say here is going to change your motivation for long.

Instead, results will be your motivation. Behavior that gets rewarded gets repeated, especially when it comes at a low cost.

Other fitness programs would have you climbing a mountain just to see results. They have you doing way more than you need to. When you factor in all the money and time other programs require, ultimately, most people decide subconsciously those costs are just too high for the rewards they reap, and they stop working out.

But this book offers you the distilled results of me spending a lifetime getting you the most meaningful rewards as quickly as possible, without wasted effort, and that's what really drives motivation.

OBSTACLES

The three primary reasons people don't work out:

1. **I do not have time.**
2. **I do not want to pay for equipment or gym memberships.**
3. **I do not have enough space.**

Strong and Lean crushes these concerns.

We can all make time for nine minutes. I know a truck driver who pulls over and throws down a camping mat at a rest stop once a day, and ten minutes later is driving off. And the minutes you take to do these exercises a few times a week will make everything else faster and more efficient.

INJURIES: If paraplegics can run marathons and enter jujitsu contests, past injuries are not much of an excuse.

LIFE: I realize this might sound harsh, but tragedy strikes us all. You can't let it get in the way of your long-term health. For instance, I have friends who have used the loss of a parent as an excuse to stop working out. Obviously, the loss of a loved one can be absolutely devastating, and they will be missed the rest of our lives. But is there any way to disgrace your parent's memory more than having their child fall apart because they inevitably die? And building a better body also rebuilds your spirits.

Quit once and you'll be far more likely to do it again. Likewise, every time you push the excuses aside, your body and your resolve strengthen. Winning becomes a habit. As does brushing off failure and starting again.

Picking up this book may be the hardest part of my workout program. Once you get going, that's the easier part. And results become the ultimate motivator—the curves of growing muscles, a hardness you didn't have before. You'll start to look better, and you'll always continue to. You will attain the figure you desire. How long it takes to get there, though . . . naturally, that depends on how far away you are. But you will get there. And your body will feel amazing in proper alignment, moving with ease, pain-free, straight, and balanced. Once you've felt that, it's hard to go back to anything else. Because you know there exist very few priorities in life that should come above your own health and looks.

WHEN YOU LOSE TO YOUR EXCUSES:	WHEN YOU TAKE CONTROL:
You suffer bad moods, anxiety, tension, boredom, depression, insomnia, poor libido, weakness, back pain, low bone density, arthritis, immobility, heart disease, diabetes, obesity, a second-rate life	You become stronger, leaner, look better, feel better, have increased energy, and have less stress and improved self-esteem

No one but you will create time for you to work out. *There will never be the "perfect" time and condition to do a workout.* You have to create it, just as we all create a hundred excuses not to work out. But later will never be easier than now.

Right here, right now, this is *your* time. The world can wait nine minutes.

DON'T LOOK AT THE SCALE

Make performance-related goals, not weight-related ones. It's all about body composition. *Not* weight. You will be replacing fat with muscle. Muscle is smaller but heavier. So a scale reflects progress poorly, especially in females, whose weight can fluctuate by six pounds daily due to factors like water retention. A better way to judge progress is noticing how your clothes fit differently. And people, too, will notice, whether they tell you or not.

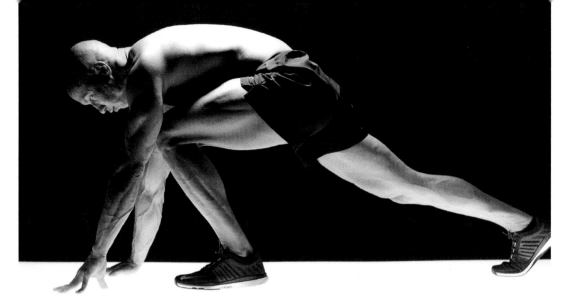

SKILL = PHYSIQUE

The athletes I've worked with have incredible physiques not because they can throw heavier weights around than you but because they're skilled at performing movements properly and efficiently. They perfectly balance stability and mobility, only moving the body parts that need to be moved while not moving the other parts.

No matter what you consider your current fitness level, everyone will see gains from following the *Strong and Lean* program from day one. You'll simply vary the number of reps you can accomplish in the time allotted. Being good at other exercises will not ensure you can plow through these movements. Performing them perfectly requires *skill* to build the best physique. It will give gym hunks and hunkettes even more desirable proportions. It will also vastly strengthen and tone newcomers to fitness. And it will help those looking to lose weight to shed those unwanted pounds. You'll be astonished how quickly you can progress to advanced levels.

ONE STEP AT A TIME

Other than the first day, you'll never have to learn more than one movement on any given day. And as the workouts progress, I'll be adding simple tips, one at a time, to ensure you're doing them with perfect form. All you need to do is turn the page.

TOTAL FITNESS, NO LIMITS, IN NINE MINUTES

The objective is achieving your best body through efficient locomotion, which requires the ability to move your arms and legs around a neutral and stable spine. That's why most days you'll first use a floor exercise to stabilize your spine. You're then challenged to move your arms and legs around that stable spine with four points of contact on the ground. Lastly, after being prepared by the floor and mobility exercises, we challenge you to put it all together where it counts most, which is in the standing exercises.

With each progression from simple to complex, you improve your posture and strengthen your ability to position yourself. These dynamic movements engage your whole body, rather than isolating tiny areas (and thus building improper proportions) and negating somewhat important things like, say, your spine.

These exercises have the added benefit of being much more demanding of core strength (*six-pack, anyone?*) than exercises that require weights and machines. They give you more strength, flexibility, and endurance while reducing the energy you need to get through life.

I've meticulously engineered every full-body workout here. Each exercise is preparing you for the next. Each nine-minute workout day is also preparing you for the next.

I've distilled it down to nine minutes, progressing from three to five times a week, in six-week cycles.

THE BIG 3

The movements are split into the Big 3:

FLOOR EXERCISES ▪ MOBILITY EXERCISES ▪ STANDING EXERCISES

These are the three categories that systematically develop your best athletic ability (which alone produces your best body). Each workout includes exercises from each of these categories, ensuring every nine-minutes trains your entire body top to bottom.

The program is broken up into six-week cycles. Just as each day builds on the last, each cycle builds more strength and skills than the last. You begin with cycle 1 and progress all the way up to cycle 4. After that, you can repeat cycles 3 and 4 endlessly. You'll still be making gains because you'll be able to do more and more reps of each exercise.

It's in the third six-week training cycle that we add nine new exercises for pushing, pulling, and hip-hinging exercises.

Lastly, we have warm-up and cool ps are made up of four exercises, the first ove hips, spine, and shoulder functi etches and relaxes you.

After your q -minute sets for each of three exercis h progression, consistency, and var s to make you stronger.

Actually, i se workouts start with 40/20 intervals l then rest for twenty seconds. You'll t -minute work intervals with no rest ase in your percentage of work time.

Remember, y cost far more than the reward. With lities you need to excel in life and loo

THE ES

Another advantage of g us. We remove the pressure to lift more or fast nally safe to perform safely.

But when I sent tra ers my exercises ahead of my earliest certification courses, some told me they found them easy! I thought, *Yikes, I must be getting old! I find these tough!* Then I'd show up and they'd proudly crank out reps for me . . . with poor posture. When I corrected them, it drastically changed the difficulty of the movements and the benefits they reaped. As I've seen again and again, even the seemingly simplest exercise is difficult if done with perfect form.

As any jujitsu master will tell you, learn just a few fundamental holds perfectly, and no one will ever be able to defeat you. This is a primary reason people spend far too long working out, not getting the results they want—because their posture is not perfect. Remember, performance is efficiency. It's amazing how little you need to do to achieve your best body, *if* you do it with perfect posture. I cannot emphasize this enough.

When I was training with my dear friend Raphael Ruiz—strength and conditioning coach to world-champion boxers, Hall of Famers in multiple sports, and Olympians who have racked up more than twenty gold medals—he always drilled into his students that posture and ideal joint alignment determine performance in all we do.

This is often the *only* reason fitness authors have better bodies than their readers. Because the authors themselves perform with perfect posture.

FOUR THINGS THAT NEVER CHANGE

As you'll see, different movements require different positions to build true strength. But these four habits *always* apply to get you into ideal alignment:

1. **Keep your feet parallel to each other. Make sure your toes do not point out at all. Imagine a line going from the *center of your heel* to the *center of all five toes.* Place your feet so these lines run parallel. This may feel strange at first, but it's vital to proper alignment.**

2. **Keep your knees pointing in the same direction as your toes.**

(These two control your hips, ensuring they are neutrally rotated, meaning neither externally rotated nor internally rotated, which is essential to safe and efficient locomotion.)

3. **When your legs are elevated, fully dorsiflex your ankles (pull your feet and toes toward your face).**

(This allows you to more easily see whether or not your feet are parallel. It also strengthens your shin muscles while improving ankle mobility.)

4. **Maintain a long, neutral spine.**

(A neutral spine is in the middle, neither flexed nor extended.)

Don't worry, we'll get you into correct posture step by step. You'll soon have an intuitive understanding of where the middle is and how to get there.

KNEES WERE MADE TO KNEEL

It's fine to use a yoga mat. But I'm finding more and more of my readers don't need them. I personally use the polished concrete floor in my condo. Because knees were made to kneel.

So why, then, does simply kneeling on a hard surface hurt so many of us? Because unlike our ancestors, we've grown so unused to doing something so vital and functional as kneeling, that when we do kneel, often our knees crash down into the floor.

But when you kneel properly, you engage all your leg muscles to control the motion, to bring your kneecap down gently. This builds and tones not only all your leg muscles but your core. It's also one of the secrets to eradicating knee pain (along with keeping your feet perfectly parallel when applicable).

THE ADVANTAGES OF A BOOK

1. A key to your success with any program is truly understanding the "why" behind it. Proper execution comes from understanding why each movement and each detail is imperative.

2. Just turn the page each day to your next workout. No navigating web pages or flipping back and forth like with other books. If it's a nine-minute workout, I don't want you spending another nine minutes trying to figure out how to execute it.

3. For the rest of your life, you have ninety-two workouts at your fingertips that can be done offline, anywhere, anytime!

4. But now you also have an exclusive invitation to stay connected via our Bodyweight Training Community at marklauren.com/strongandlean. We interact daily to answer questions, share experiences, and post fun challenges to make you healthier and happier. To enter the exclusive Strong and Lean "room," use code word *LOCOMOTION* when prompted.

Bodyweight exercises were a fitness revolution.

This is their final evolution.

Strong and Lean distills the skills it takes to achieve an athlete's body down to their most efficient form for the first time in history. You're holding the double-edged sword—a program that gains you the *quickest* beach body results through movements that lead to *lifelong* athleticism. You're going to learn to move and shape your body like a lean, muscled athlete, because you will be one.

THE *STRONG AND LEAN* PROGRAM

The days of the week here are suggestions. If you need to alter them because of your schedule, that's okay. But it's crucial you stick to a schedule.

OVERVIEW

For a bird's eye view of this program, download the Exercise Matrix and Training Schedules at marklauren.com/strongandlean.

TIMER

These workouts require a timer. If you don't have one, I have custom-made nine-minute timers for you at marklauren.com/strongandlean. I made a simple video timer that you can download to your phone. Save it to your favorites and hit Play when you're ready to train. A second timer is available to you on the Strong and Lean page that also walks you through the warm ups.

Share your journey with us on Instagram! Post a pic of yourself with the hashtag #9minuteworkouts and tag us @mark_lauren_training.

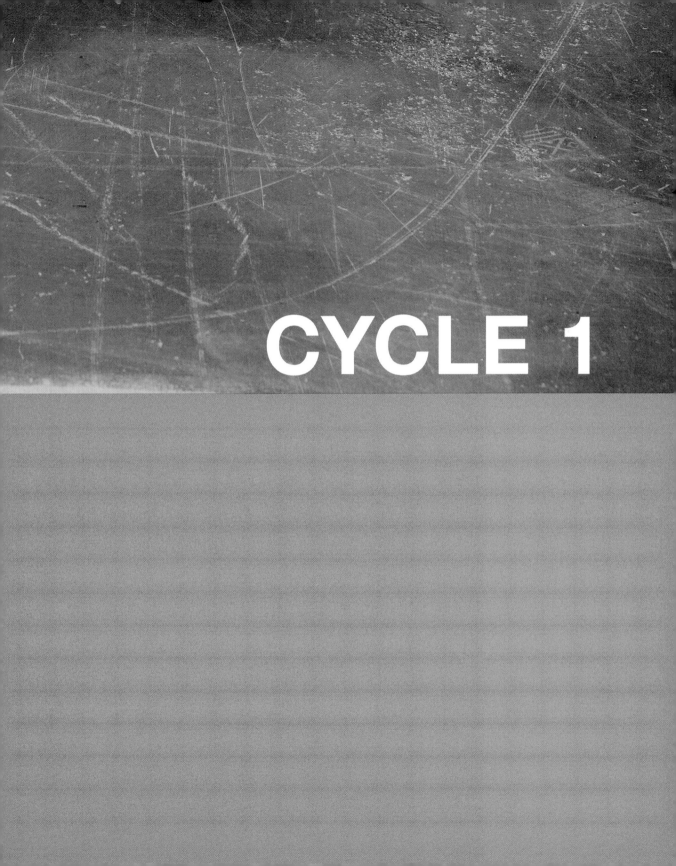

CYCLE 1

Warm-ups are made up of four exercises, the first to get your heart rate up and the other three to improve hips, spine, and shoulder functions. Cool-downs are made up of a single exercise that stretches and relaxes you. These only take a minute.

WARM-UP

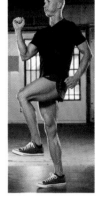

To kick things off, let's get your heart rate up by marching in place for sixty seconds. Take it nice and easy. Focus on your posture, breathing, and rhythm.

Then do two rounds of eight easy reps of each of these:

HIP CIRCLES

Open up your hips and activate your glutes

Get into a crawling position with your hips over your knees and your shoulders over your wrists. Keeping your left knee bent at ninety degrees, slightly raise the left leg off the floor. Then make eight giant circles going backward. At the top of the circle, get your knee up as high as you can. Control the movement and don't swing your leg. Do eight reps on the left side and eight reps on the right side. Then repeat for two rounds total.

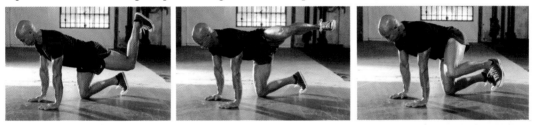

TWIST AND REACH

Improve your shoulder and thoracic spine mobility

From a crawling position, reach your left arm under your body to the right side, and then reach up as high as you can while pushing the supporting arm into the floor to make yourself as big as possible at the top of the movement. Exhale as you reach up. Do eight reps on the left side and eight reps on the right side. Then repeat for two rounds total.

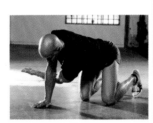
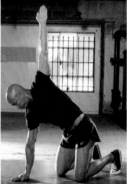

POINTERS

Flexion and extension of the hips, spine, and shoulders

From a crawling position, bring your left elbow to your right knee. Then extend both your left arm and right leg upward until your back is arched. Exhale as you reach up. Perform eight reps and then switch sides. Then repeat for two rounds total.

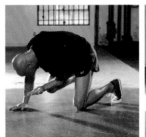
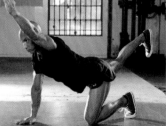

WORKOUT

**DO EACH EXERCISE FOR JUST FORTY SECONDS,
FOLLOWED BY TWENTY SECONDS OF REST.**

PARALLEL LEG CRUNCH

Abs, hip flexors, obliques, neck, deltoids, shin muscles, quadriceps, hip rotators, rib muscles, traps

Lie down on your back with your legs elevated and your hips, knees, and ankles bent at ninety degrees. Don't cross your ankles.

INHALE: Reach up with both arms as high as you can. Try to touch the sky.
EXHALE: Lower yourself slowly, bringing your arms down to the Y position. At the bottom of the movement, reach past your head to the Y position as far as possible while keeping your lower back in contact with the floor and blowing out all your air.

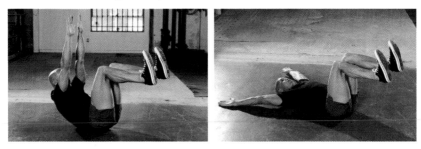

STARFISH TWIST

Deltoids, triceps, forearms, lats, spinal erectors, abs, obliques, rib muscles, hip flexors, glutes, shin muscles, calves, hamstrings, quadriceps, hip abductors/adductors, pectorals, biceps, neck

Get into the starting position of a Push-Up with your wrists underneath your shoulders. Place your feet hip-width apart! This is important, so you can roll your heels without bumping into your feet.

INHALE: Roll your heels all the way to the left.
EXHALE: Reach your right arm straight up to the sky and get into a side planking position.
INHALE: While keeping your right arm raised, rotate your hips so they are parallel to the floor again. **The key here is to rotate the hips independently of the shoulders.**
EXHALE: Once you've rolled onto the balls of your feet again, bring your right arm down to the starting position of a Push-Up.

Repeat on the opposite side.

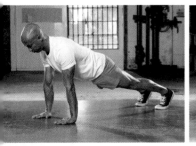
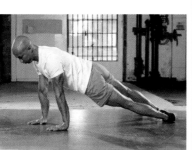
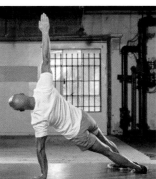
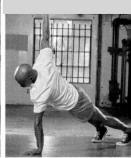

STORK STANCE

Glutes, hip abductors/adductors, hamstrings, quadriceps, calves, hip flexors, abs, obliques, spinal erectors, deltoids, shin muscles, hip rotators, lats, traps

Start in a tall double kneeling position with your arms at the T position.

INHALE: Step forward with your left leg into a long single kneeling position.
EXHALE: Stand up on your left leg and pull your right knee up.
INHALE: Reverse the movement to get back into a long single kneeling position with your left leg forward.
EXHALE: Transition to a tall double kneeling position.

Switch sides after each rep.

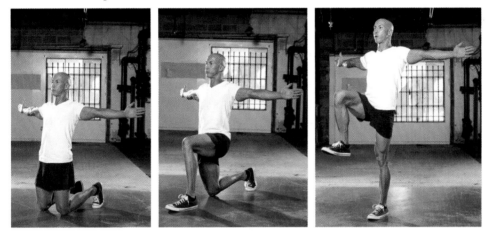

COOL-DOWN

A-FRAMES *(six slow reps each side)*

Stretch the calves, hamstrings, hips, and lats

Get into the starting position of a Push-Up, and place your left foot next to your left hand.

Straighten your left leg, and pull the toes of your left foot up toward your face until you feel a stretch in your left calf and hamstring.

Return to the starting position, and then lower your left forearm to the floor to stretch your left hip.

Take your time, relax, and get at least one full breath in each position. Perform six reps, and then switch sides.

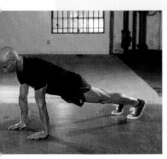
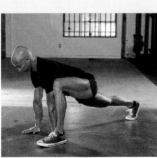
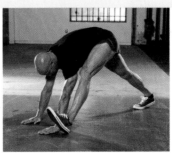
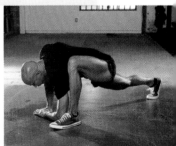

WARM-UP

March in Place (for sixty seconds)

Then do eight reps of each of these exercises, for two rounds total:

HIP CIRCLES   TWIST AND REACH   POINTERS

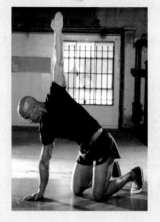
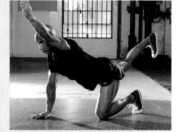

WORKOUT

40/20 WORK-TO-REST INTERVALS.

PARALLEL LEG BRIDGE

Glutes, hamstrings, abs, shin muscles, spinal erectors, lats, traps, deltoids, forearms

Lie on your back with your arms at your sides, palms up. Pull your feet to your butt, and place them flat on the floor, hip-width apart. Your knees should be bent and pointing straight up, your legs parallel.

EXHALE: Raise your hips as high as you can. Make yourself straight from your knees to the base of your neck. Squeeze your glutes and abs at the top.
INHALE: Lower yourself.

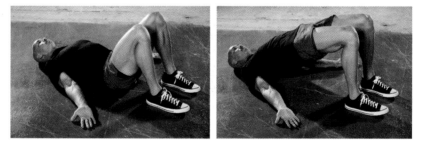

STARFISH TWIST

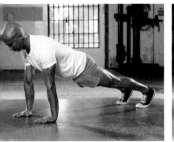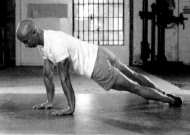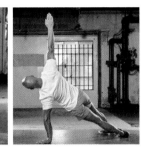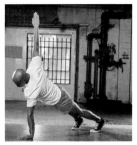

STORK STANCE

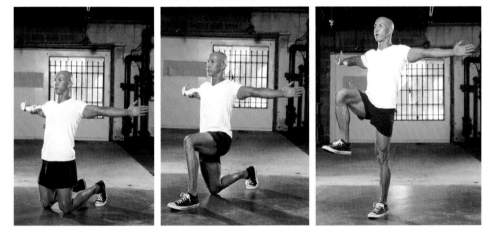

COOL-DOWN

SPIDERMAN A-FRAMES *(six slow reps each side)*

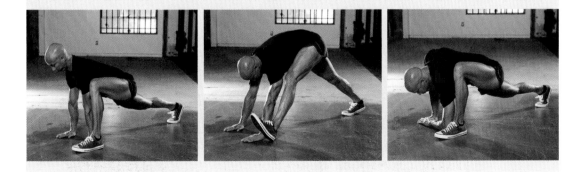

WARM-UP

March in Place (for sixty seconds)

Then do eight reps of each of these exercises, for two rounds total:

HIP CIRCLES   TWIST AND REACH   POINTERS

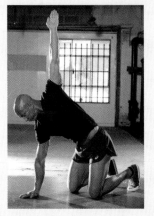
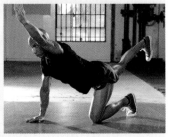

WORKOUT

40/20 WORK-TO-REST INTERVALS.

ARM HAULERS

Deltoids, rib muscles, traps, glutes, abs, neck, shin muscles, quadriceps, lats, spinal erectors, triceps, forearms

Lie on your stomach with your arms extended past your head in a long streamline position, palms down. Position your feet hip-width apart with your toes on the floor. Throughout this exercise, keep your glutes flexed, belly button sucked in, and chest on the floor.

INHALE: Swing your arms to the sides of your body as if you're trying to make a snow angel while lying on your stomach.

EXHALE: Swing your arms in a big arch back up to the streamline position. Make yourself as long as possible.

Your breathing sets the pace for this exercise, as for all others.

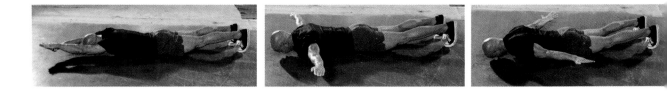

PARALLEL LEG CRUNCH

TIP: Be sure to exhale forcefully on the way down.

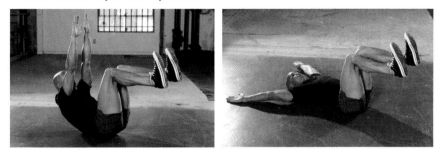

PARALLEL LEG BRIDGE

TIP: Exhale forcefully on the way up.

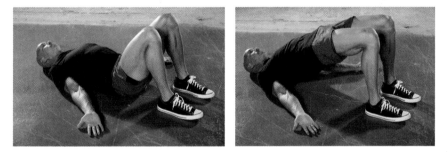

COOL-DOWN

SPIDERMAN A-FRAMES *(six slow reps each side)*

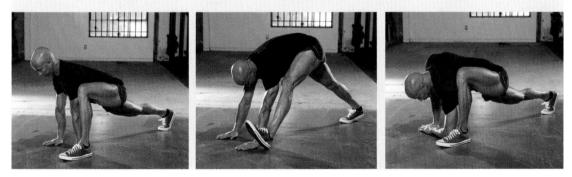

WARM-UP

March in Place (for sixty seconds)

Then do eight reps of each of these exercises, for two rounds total:

HIP CIRCLES   TWIST AND REACH   POINTERS

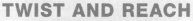

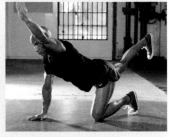

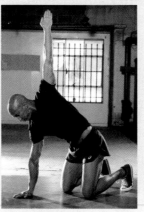

WORKOUT

40/20 WORK-TO-REST INTERVALS.

ARM HAULERS

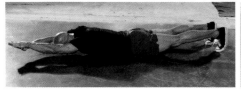

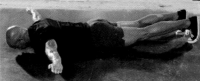

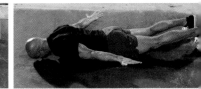

STARFISH TWIST

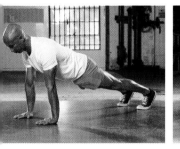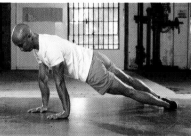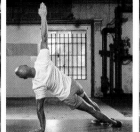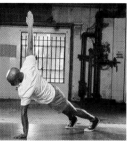

STORK STANCE

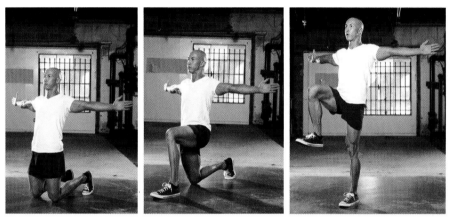

COOL-DOWN

SPIDERMAN ARM CIRCLES *(eight reps each side)*

Improved hip, spine, and shoulder mobility

From the starting position of a Push-Up, place your left foot next to your left hand.

EXHALE: Raise your left hand off the floor and make a giant circle with your left arm. Keep your eyes on your left hand as you place the knuckles of your left hand on your lower back.
INHALE: Reverse the movement.

Keep your hips low and your lead knee pointing straight ahead throughout this exercise.

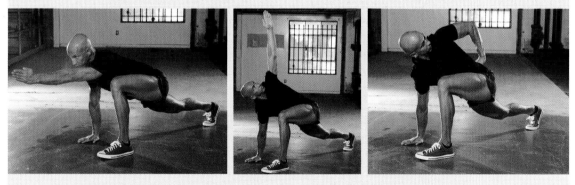

WARM-UP

March in Place (for sixty seconds)

Then do eight reps of each of these exercises, for two rounds total:

HIP CIRCLES   TWIST AND REACH   POINTERS

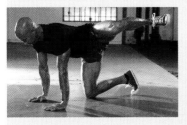
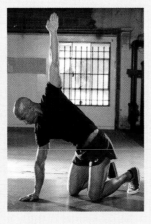
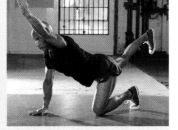

WORKOUT

40/20 WORK-TO-REST INTERVALS.

PARALLEL LEG BRIDGE

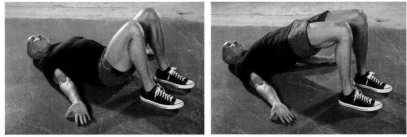

STARFISH TWIST

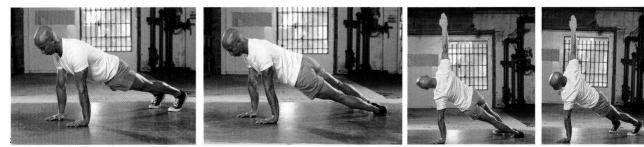

BOTTOM SQUAT

Shin muscles, glutes, hip rotators, hip abductors/adductors, hamstrings, quadriceps, calves, obliques, spinal erectors, hip flexors, abs, lats, deltoids, traps

Start in a tall double kneeling position with your arms out to the front, zombie-style.

INHALE: Step forward with the left leg into a single kneeling position.
EXHALE: Pull the right leg into position so that you're in a Squat with your feet parallel and knees pointing straight ahead. Keep your hips low and your chest up.
INHALE: Reverse the movement by stepping back with your left leg.
EXHALE: Transition from single kneeling to double kneeling.

Lead with the right leg for the following rep. This exercise has rhythmic side-to-side weight shifting: *right, left, right, left.* For the next rep: *left, right, left, right.*

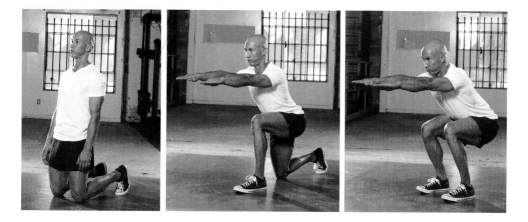

COOL-DOWN

SPIDERMAN ARM CIRCLES *(eight reps each side)*

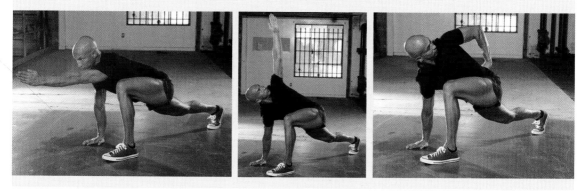

CRAWLING WARM-UP

March in Place (for sixty seconds)

Then do eight reps of each of these exercises, for two rounds total:

HIP CIRCLES TWIST AND REACH POINTERS

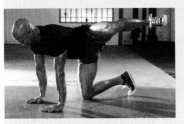
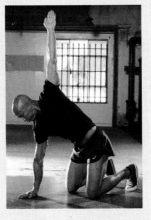
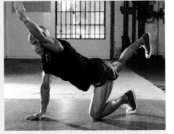

WORKOUT

40/20 WORK-TO-REST INTERVALS.

ARM HAULERS

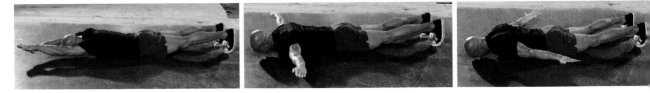

LOW DROP

Deltoids, triceps, lats, spinal erectors, abs, obliques, rib muscles, hip flexors, glutes, shin muscles, calves, hamstrings, quadriceps, hip abductors/adductors, pectorals, biceps, forearms, neck

Start in a planking position on your forearms. Place your feet hip-width apart.

Roll your heels all the way to the left, and transition to a left-side planking position with your right arm on your hips.

INHALE: Lower your hips to the floor.
EXHALE: Raise them.

Transition back to a planking position on both forearms before switching sides.

Make yourself straight in the side planking positions: Tense your glutes, lift your chest slightly, tighten your abs, and check the position of your head. Hold that posture as you transition from side to side.

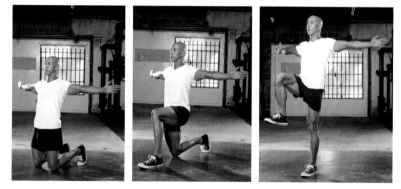

STORK STANCE

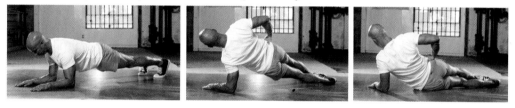

COOL-DOWN
SPIDERMAN ARM CIRCLES *(eight reps each side)*

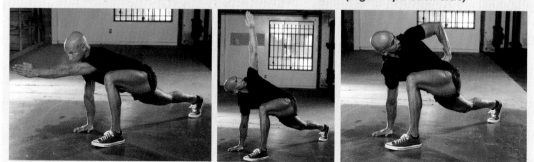

CRAWLING WARM-UP

March in Place (for sixty seconds)

Then do eight reps of each of these exercises, for two rounds total:

HIP CIRCLES   TWIST AND REACH   POINTERS

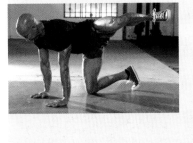
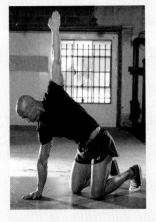
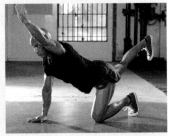

WORKOUT

NOW DO EACH EXERCISE FOR FORTY-FIVE SECONDS, FOLLOWED BY FIFTEEN SECONDS OF REST.

PARALLEL LEG CRUNCH

TIPS: Fully flex both ankles so that you're pulling your toes back toward your face and keeping your feet parallel to each other. This improves ankle mobility and your ability to control hip rotation, which will improve your alignment for standing exercises so you can safely absorb the stress needed to stay strong and lean long-term.

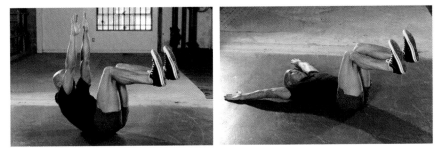

STARFISH TWIST

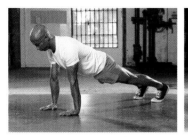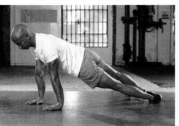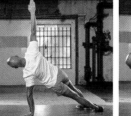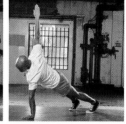

HIGH-KNEE MARCH

Shin muscles, glutes, hip flexors, hip rotators, hamstrings, quadriceps, calves, abs, obliques, spinal erectors, deltoids, lats, traps, hip abductors/adductors, biceps, neck

March in Place. Stand up tall and straight, keep your feet parallel, and find a steady pace. Get your knees up high, and use a strong arm swing while keeping your elbows bent at ninety degrees.

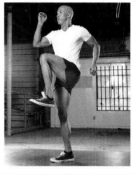

COOL-DOWN

BLOOMERS *(eight slow reps)*

Stretch the back of your body and improve shoulder mobility

Stand with your feet parallel to each other and hip-width apart. Keep your legs straight throughout this exercise.

Bend over at the waist, and let your upper body, arms, and head hang straight down. Try to relax. Come to a complete and relaxed hang.

Suck in your belly button, and slowly roll yourself back up to a tall standing position.

Then perform a big arm swing to the streamline position while exhaling fully. Make yourself tall.

Get a big arm swing on the way down and lead with your head as you roll yourself down, sucking in your belly button.

Feel the stretch along your spine as you roll yourself up and down. Do eight slow and controlled reps.

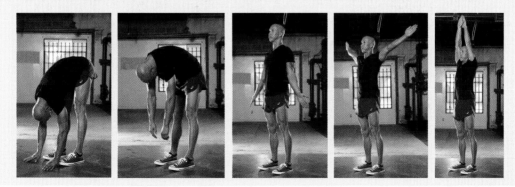

CRAWLING WARM-UP

March in Place (for sixty seconds)

Then do eight reps of each of these exercises, for two rounds total:

HIP CIRCLES   TWIST AND REACH   POINTERS

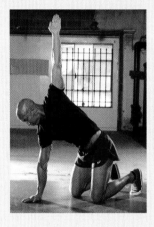
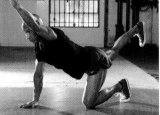

45/15 WORK-TO-REST INTERVALS.

PARALLEL LEG BRIDGE

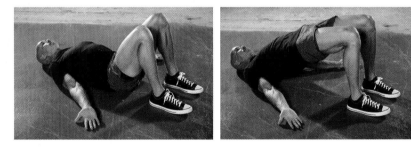

LOW DROP

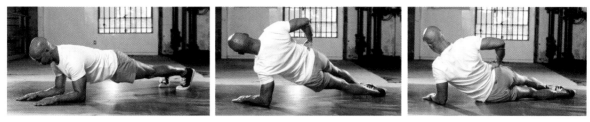

HIGH-KNEE MARCH

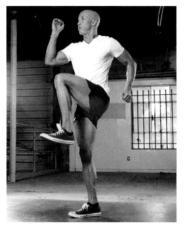

COOL-DOWN

BLOOMERS *(eight slow reps)*

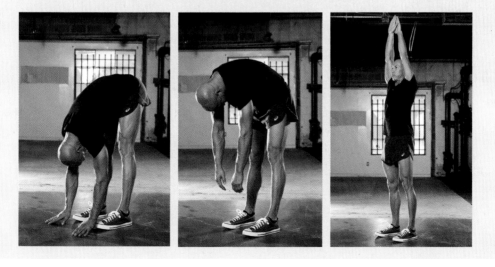

CRAWLING WARM-UP

March in Place (for sixty seconds)

Then do eight reps of each of these exercises, for two rounds total:

HIP CIRCLES   TWIST AND REACH   POINTERS

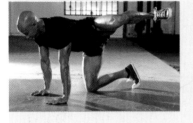 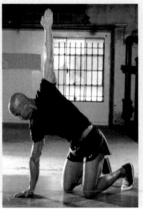 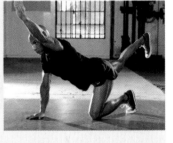

WORKOUT

45/15 WORK-TO-REST INTERVALS.

ARM HAULERS

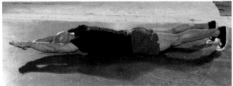 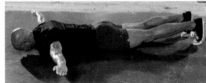 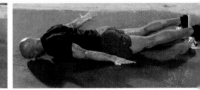

KICKOUT

Deltoids, triceps, forearms, abs, hip flexors, obliques, spinal erectors, lats, quadriceps, shin muscles, calves, hamstrings, glutes, internal hip rotators, rib muscles, traps, neck

Start in a crawling position with your hands a couple of inches in front of your knees. Elevate your knees off the floor slightly.

INHALE: Rotate your knees to the left about forty-five degrees, and then raise your left hand and right foot off the floor.

EXHALE: Continue rotating until you are able to fully extend the right leg in front of you.

In the Kickout position, point the toes and knee of the extended leg straight up to the sky. Let your hips rest on your supporting leg and lift your chest slightly. Make it look good!

Reset to the starting position with your knees close to your hands, and switch sides.

Don't rush. Focus on transitioning smoothly and getting into the perfect end position.

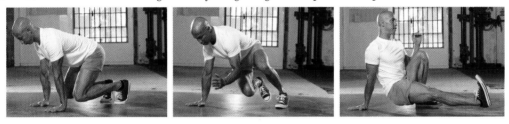

BOTTOM SQUAT

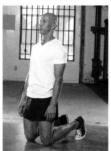
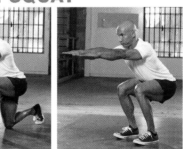

COOL-DOWN

BLOOMERS *(eight slow reps)*

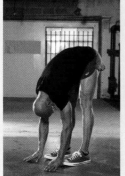
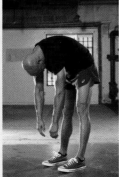
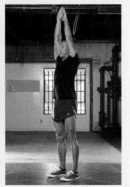

CRAWLING WARM-UP

March in Place (for sixty seconds)

Then do eight reps of each of these exercises, for two rounds total:

HIP CIRCLES   TWIST AND REACH   POINTERS

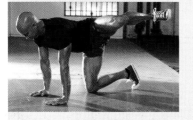
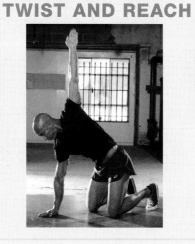
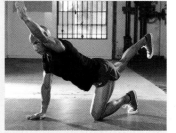

WORKOUT

45/15 WORK-TO-REST INTERVALS.

PARALLEL LEG CRUNCH

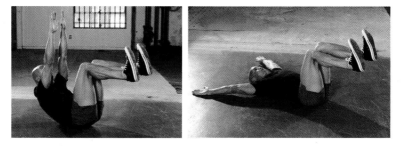

PARALLEL LEG BRIDGE

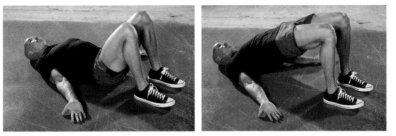

ARM HAULERS

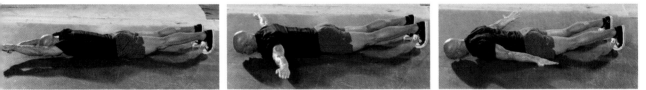

COOL-DOWN

STRADDLE REACH *(eight reps each side)*

Stretch your inner thighs and lats

Sit on the floor and spread your legs until you feel a light stretch in your inner thighs. Dorsiflex both ankles, and keep your toes and knees pointing straight up.

Reach both arms up to a tall streamline position while exhaling. Lift your chest slightly.

Then place your left hand on the floor behind your back, and reach toward or past your left foot with your right hand, rounding your back slightly for a full stretch. Hold the position for a full exhalation.

Then reach to the streamline position again, before reaching to the right foot with the left hand.

Take your time and exhale as you reach to each of the positions.

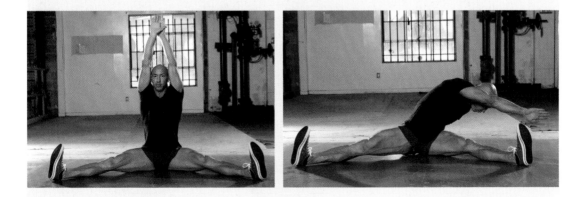

CRAWLING WARM-UP

March in Place (for sixty seconds)

Then do eight reps of each of these exercises, for two rounds total:

HIP CIRCLES   TWIST AND REACH   POINTERS

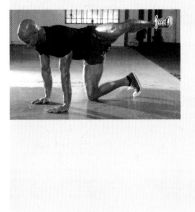
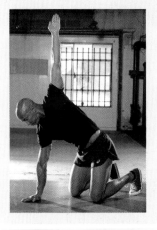
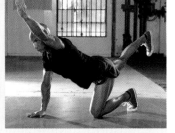

WORKOUT

45/15 WORK-TO-REST INTERVALS.

BENT LEG BRIDGE

Glutes, hamstrings, hip flexors, abs, shin muscles, obliques, spinal erectors, lats, lower/mid traps, deltoids, forearms

Lie on your back with your arms at your sides, palms up. Pull your feet to your butt, and place them flat on the floor, hip-width apart. Your knees should be bent and pointing straight up. Pull your right knee into your chest.

EXHALE: Raise your hips up as high as you can, flexing your abdominals at the top.
INHALE: Lower your hips.

Repeat for two reps, then switch legs.

Keep the knee of the elevated leg actively pulled into your chest as you raise and lower your hips.

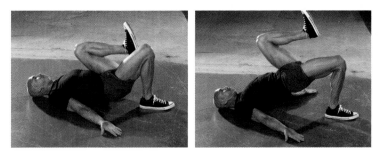

STARFISH TWIST

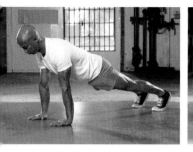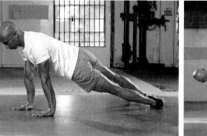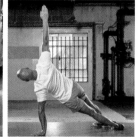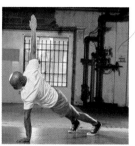

BOTTOM SQUAT

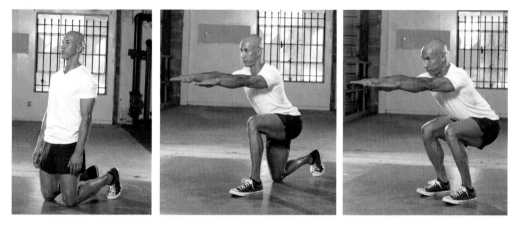

COOL-DOWN

STRADDLE REACH *(eight reps each side)*

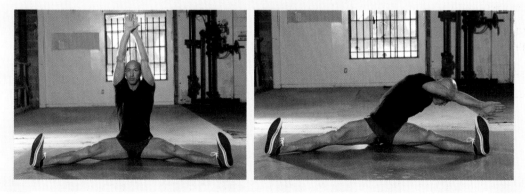

CRAWLING WARM-UP

March in Place (for sixty seconds)

Then do eight reps of each of these exercises, for two rounds total:

HIP CIRCLES   TWIST AND REACH   POINTERS

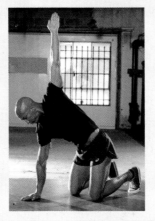
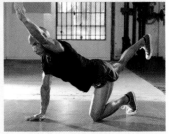

WORKOUT

45/15 WORK-TO-REST INTERVALS.

ARM HAULERS

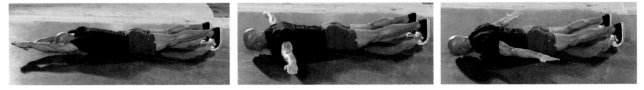

LOW DROP

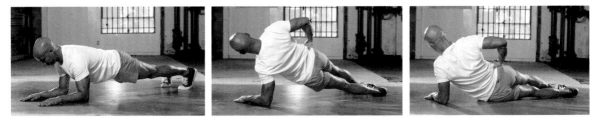

STREAMLINE ROMANIAN DEAD LIFT

Glutes, hamstrings, quadriceps, lats, traps, spinal erectors, shin muscles, deltoids, calves, abs, triceps, forearms, neck

Stand tall with your feet parallel and shoulder-width apart. Raise your arms up to the streamline position.

INHALE: While keeping your legs straight, push your hips back and let your upper body tilt forward with a straight back until you feel a stretch in your hamstrings. Go down only as far as you can with a straight back! Once you feel a stretch in your hamstrings, don't go down any farther. Instead, take a moment to push your hips back while reaching your arms past your head as far as you can. Make yourself as long as possible.

EXHALE: Reverse the movement, and reset to a tall standing position.

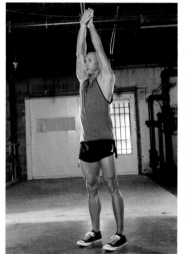
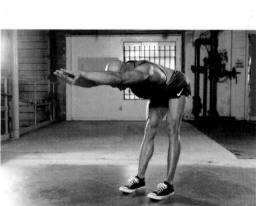

COOL-DOWN

STRADDLE REACH *(eight reps each side)*

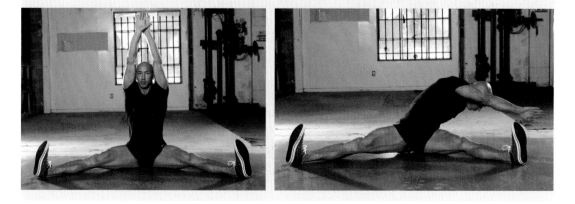

CRAWLING WARM-UP

March in Place (for sixty seconds)

Then do eight reps of each of these exercises, for two rounds total:

HIP CIRCLES   TWIST AND REACH   POINTERS

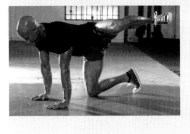 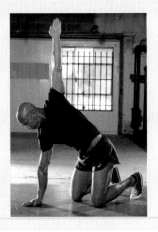 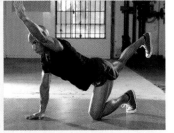

WORKOUT

50/10 WORK-TO-REST INTERVALS.

PARALLEL LEG CRUNCH

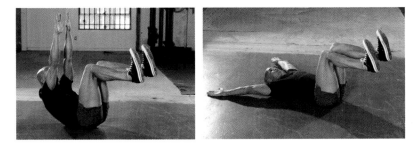

KICKOUT

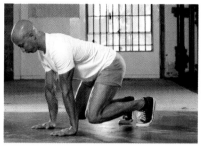 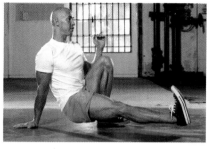

HIGH-KNEE MARCH

TIP: With each step, fully extend through the supporting leg while lifting your chest slightly and keeping your abs tensed. Get your knees up and swing your arms with your elbows bent at ninety degrees. This basic movement pattern has a lot of useful carry over to real-life activities when done properly.

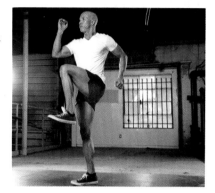

COOL-DOWN

ISOMETRIC PIGEON STRETCH *(8 x 10 seconds on each side)*

Stretch your hip flexors and glutes

Position your left leg in front of you with your left shin perpendicular to your body, or as close to perpendicular as you can get it without much effort. If your left shin is nowhere close to being perpendicular, don't worry. That's what we're working toward. Your right leg should be fully extended behind you with your right knee pointing straight down.

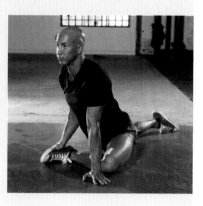

Place the left hand directly in front of the left knee, and pin your left foot to the floor using your right hand. Push your left ankle into the floor for ten seconds.

Relax and instantly sink your hips farther toward the floor while moving your hips away from your foot, millimeter by millimeter.

Repeat eight times and then switch sides.

CRAWLING WARM-UP

March in Place (for sixty seconds)

Then do eight reps of each of these exercises, for two rounds total:

HIP CIRCLES   TWIST AND REACH   POINTERS

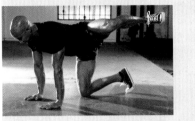
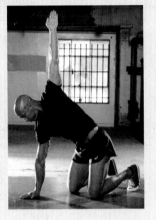
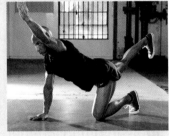

WORKOUT

50/10 WORK-TO-REST INTERVALS.

BENT LEG BRIDGE

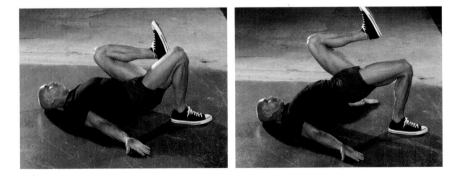

Y CUFF

Deltoids, rib muscles, shoulder rotators, traps, shin muscles, quadriceps, glutes, abs, spinal erectors, lats, neck, triceps, forearms

In a front lying position, keep your feet parallel and hip-width apart with your toes on the floor. Flex your glutes, draw in your navel, and keep your chest on the floor with your chin slightly tucked.

Fully extend your arms to the Y position, thumbs up.

INHALE: Pull your hands under your armpits, and straighten your arms at your sides, so that your fingers are pointing toward your feet. Your palms should be facing outward, thumbs up.

EXHALE: Turn your palms toward one another, and then keep turning until your thumbs are pointing up again.

INHALE: Reverse the rotation.

EXHALE: Pull your hands under your armpits again to reset them to the Y position.

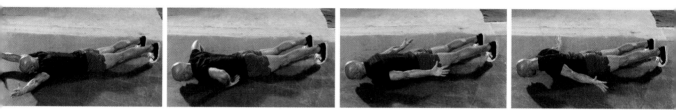

PARALLEL LEG CRUNCH

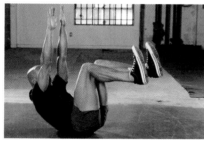 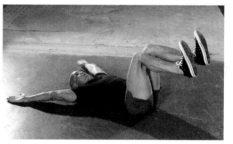

COOL-DOWN
ISOMETRIC PIGEON STRETCH

(8 x 10 seconds on each side)

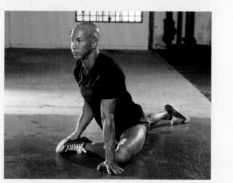

CRAWLING WARM-UP

March in Place (for sixty seconds)

Then do eight reps of each of these exercises, for two rounds total:

HIP CIRCLES   TWIST AND REACH   POINTERS

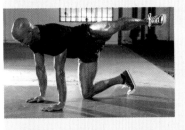
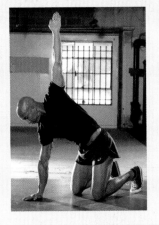
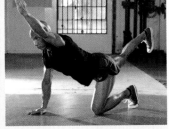

WORKOUT

50/10 WORK-TO-REST INTERVALS.

ARM HAULERS

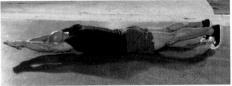
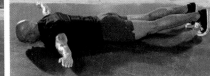
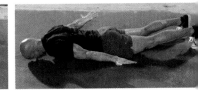

STARFISH TWIST

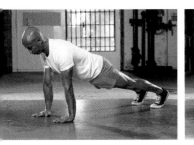
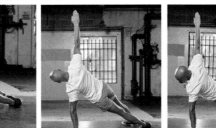
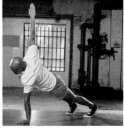

T-ARM SQUAT

Glutes, hamstrings, quadriceps, lats, traps, spinal erectors, shin muscles, calves, hip rotators, abs, neck, deltoids

Get into a tall standing position with your feet parallel and shoulder-width apart. Extend your arms out fully to the T position.

INHALE: Push your hips straight back and let your hips sink as far as you can while keeping your chest up and knees pointing straight ahead.

EXHALE: Stand up tall and straight again, by squeezing your glutes, lifting your chest slightly, and forcefully blowing out all your air. Reset your feet to parallel, and fully straighten your arms before starting the next rep.

You'll make the best gains by taking your time and challenging your range of motion.

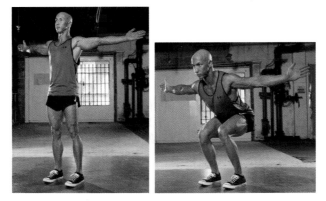

COOL-DOWN

ISOMETRIC PIGEON STRETCH
(8 x 10 seconds on each side)

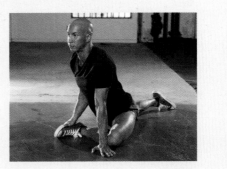

CRAWLING WARM-UP

March in Place (for sixty seconds)

Then do eight reps of each of these exercises, for two rounds total:

HIP CIRCLES   TWIST AND REACH   POINTERS

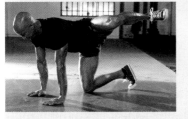
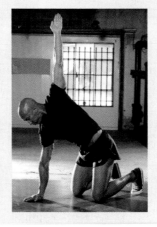
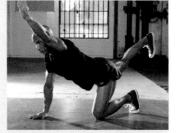

WORKOUT

50/10 WORK-TO-REST INTERVALS.

PARALLEL LEG CRUNCH

TIP: At the bottom of the movement, keep your lower back in contact with the floor. Use your abs to control your pelvic tilt and thereby the arch in your lower back. A partner should not be able to slide their hand under your lower back at any time. Learning to control pelvic tilting is essential to good posture and a healthy spine.

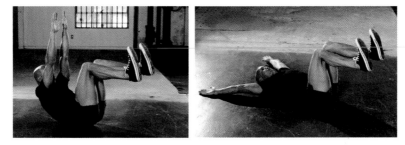

KICKOUT

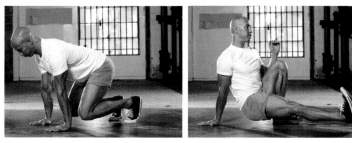

BOTTOM SQUAT

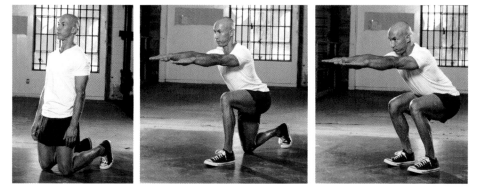

COOL-DOWN

HIP ROLLS *(eight slow reps)*

Hip and spine rotation

Lie on your back with your arms at the Y position. With ninety-degree bends in your knees, position your feet so that they're slightly wider than shoulder-width apart.

Roll your knees to the left and *gently* pull your right knee down toward the floor for a couple of breaths.

Roll your knees to the right and *gently* pull your left knee down toward the floor for a couple of breaths.

Maintain tension in your abdominals to keep your back from arching.

Perform eight reps on each side.

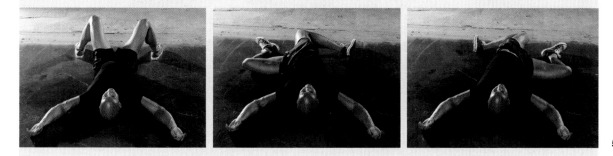

CRAWLING WARM-UP

March in Place (for sixty seconds)

Then do eight reps of each of these exercises, for two rounds total:

HIP CIRCLES   TWIST AND REACH   POINTERS

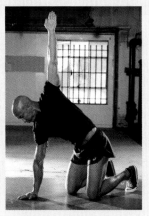
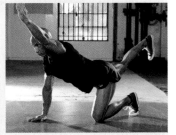

WORKOUT

50/10 WORK-TO-REST INTERVALS.

BENT LEG BRIDGE

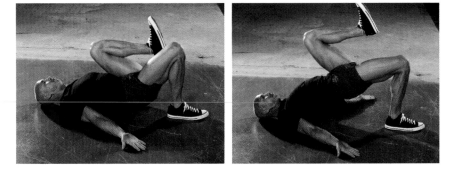

HIGH KICK

Deltoids, triceps, forearms, abs, hip flexors, obliques, spinal erectors, lats, calves, hamstrings, glutes, quadriceps, shin muscles, internal hip rotators, rib muscles, traps, neck

From the quadruped position, rotate left, and perform a Kickout with the right leg. Reset to the starting position without setting your right foot on the floor.

EXHALE: Kick the right leg straight up while extending the left leg fully and pushing your chest down toward the left foot so that your hips are raised into the air. As you straighten the supporting leg, let the heel sink to the floor to get a good stretch through your calf and hamstring.
INHALE: Lower yourself to the starting position.

Repeat on the other side.

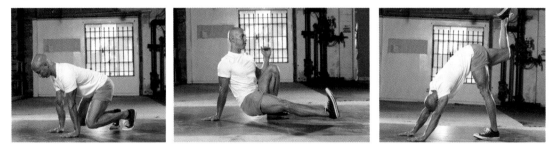

STREAMLINE ROMANIAN DEAD LIFT

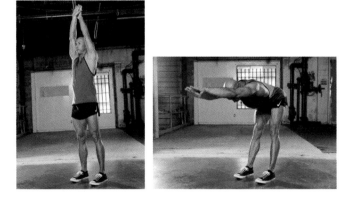

COOL-DOWN

HIP ROLLS *(eight slow reps)*

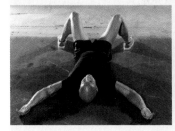 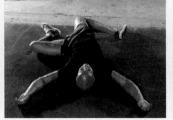 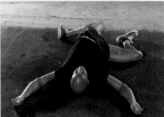

CRAWLING WARM-UP

March in Place (for sixty seconds)

Then do eight reps of each of these exercises, for two rounds total:

HIP CIRCLES TWIST AND REACH POINTERS

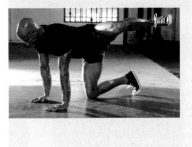
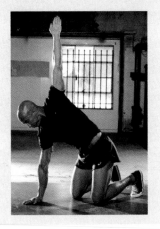
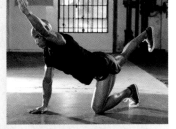

WORKOUT

50/10 WORK-TO-REST INTERVALS.

Y CUFF

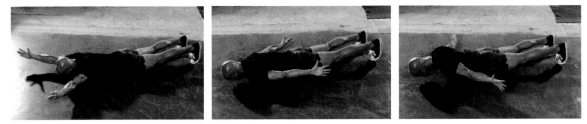

BENT LEG CRUNCH

Abs, hip flexors, obliques, neck, deltoids, shin muscles, quadriceps, glutes, hip rotators, rib muscles, traps

This exercise starts just like the Parallel Leg Crunch, with your hips, knees, and ankles bent at ninety degrees.

INHALE: Reach up to the sky.

EXHALE: Lower yourself while bringing your arms back to the Y position with your lower back flat against the floor. However, as you lower yourself, also straighten your left leg so that it comes down and to the left side.

Reset the leg as you reach up again, and then switch legs for the next rep.

Throughout this exercise, fully flex your ankles so that your toes are being pulled back toward your face. Keep your toes and knees pointing straight up as you extend your legs by internally rotating your hips.

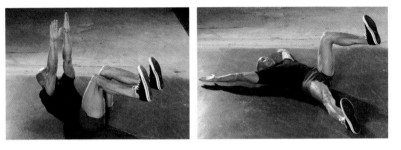

T-ARM SQUAT

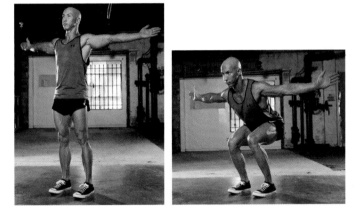

COOL-DOWN

HIP ROLLS *(eight slow reps)*

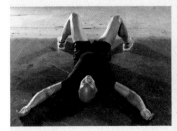 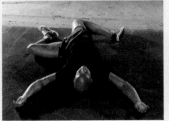 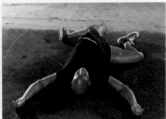

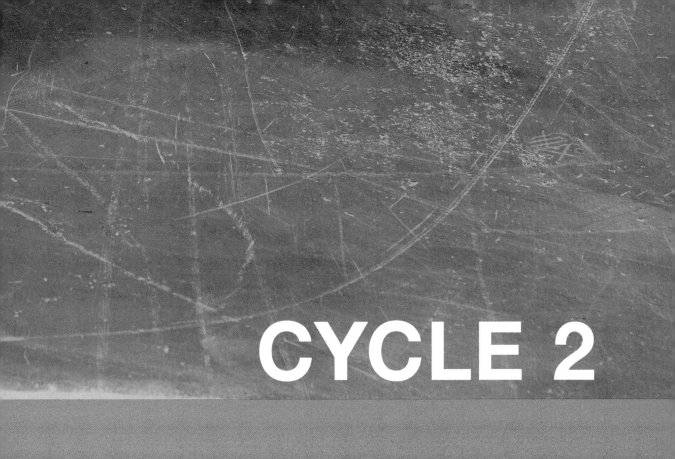

CYCLE 2

With each progression from simple to complex, you improve your posture and strengthen your ability to position yourself. These dynamic movements engage your whole body.

WARM-UP

We're starting with sixty seconds of Jumping Jacks. Your feet should remain parallel and your midsection tight so you don't arch your back as you swing your arms overhead. Stay relaxed, breathe, and focus on rhythm.

Do two rounds of the below three-exercise circuit.

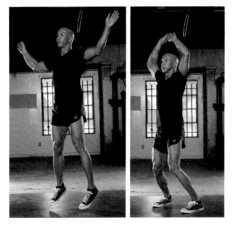

SIDE-LYING LEG LIFTS

Activate your glutes and internal hip rotators

Lie down on your left side with a long, straight body position. Cradle your head with your left arm, and place your right forearm on the floor in front of you. Raise your right leg as high as you can while keeping the right knee rotated down toward the floor. Maintain internal hip rotation while raising the top leg, so that you feel this movement in your upper glutes, not your hip flexors. Perform eight reps, and then roll onto your right side to do eight reps using the left leg. Keep the elevated ankle flexed with the toes pulled toward yourself.

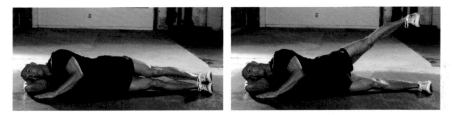

ITB LEG LIFTS

Lie on your left side. Cross your right foot over your left leg. Grab your right foot with your right hand. Internally rotate your left hip so that your left knee is fully turned up toward the sky.

While maintaining full internal hip rotation, slowly raise your leg while exhaling forcefully. Inhale as you slowly lower your leg and repeat. Keep your left knee turned straight up to the sky!

Do eight reps while lying on your left side and eight reps while lying on your right side.

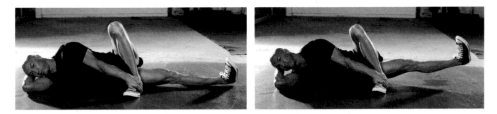

BACKSTROKE

While lying on your left side, pull your knees up toward your chest so that your hips and knees are bent at ninety degrees. Fully extend the top arm. Make eight big circles going backward. Take your time, breathe, and try to relax as you make giant circles. Keep your knees pulled up and stacked on top of each other.

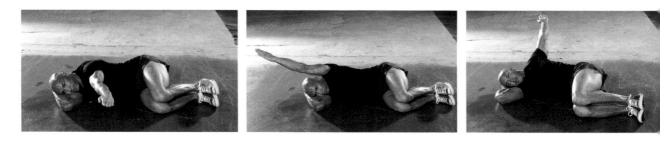

WORKOUT

40/20 WORK-TO-REST INTERVALS.

ARM HAULERS

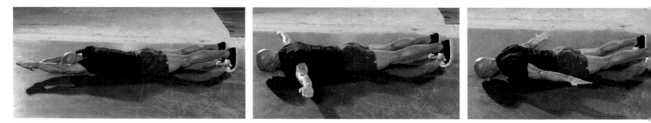

STARFISH TWIST

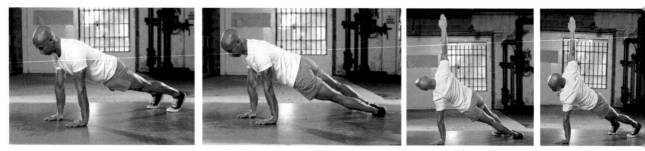

STORK STANCE

TIPS: Make yourself as tall as possible in the double kneeling, single kneeling, and standing positions. Fully extend through your hips, lift your chest, and tighten your abs as if you might get punched in the gut at any moment.

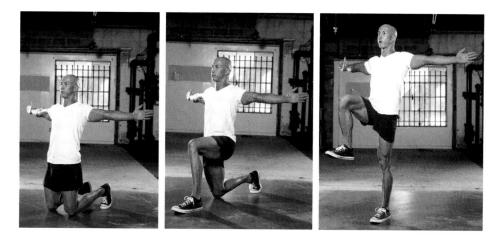

COOL-DOWN

SPIDERMAN A-FRAMES *(six slow reps each side)*

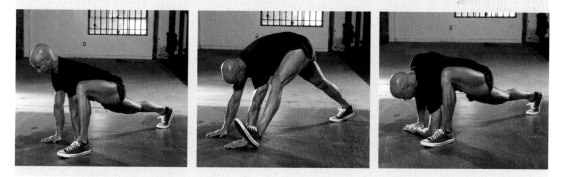

WARM-UP

Jumping Jacks (for sixty seconds)

Then do eight reps of each of these exercises, for two rounds total:

SIDE-LYING LEG LIFTS ITB LEG LIFTS BACKSTROKE

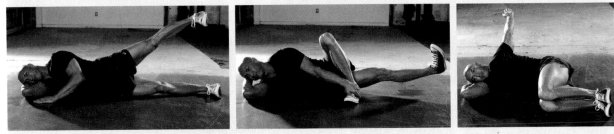

WORKOUT

40/20 WORK-TO-REST INTERVALS.

BENT LEG BRIDGE

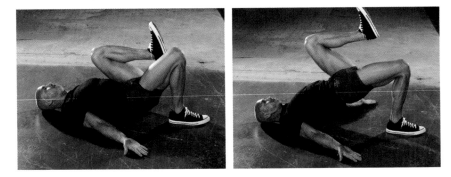

HIGH DROP

Deltoids, triceps, forearms, lats, spinal erectors, abs, obliques, rib muscles, hip flexors, glutes, shin muscles, calves, hamstrings, quadriceps, hip abductors/adductors, pectorals, biceps, neck

Get into the starting position of a Push-Up with your wrists directly underneath your shoulders. Place your feet hip-width apart so you can roll your heels to either side and transition to a side planking position without your feet bumping into each other.

Roll your heels all the way to the left. Transition to a side planking position on your left side with your right arm on your hips.

INHALE: Lower your hips to the floor.
EXHALE: Raise them.

Reset to the starting position of a Push-Up.

Switch sides.

Make yourself straight in the Push-Up and side planking positions by tensing your glutes, lifting your chest, tightening your abs, and checking the position of your head.

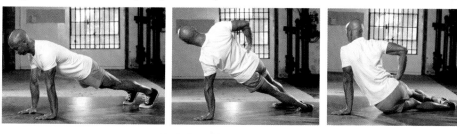

BOTTOM SQUAT

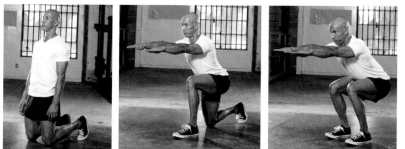

COOL-DOWN

SPIDERMAN A-FRAMES *(six slow reps each side)*

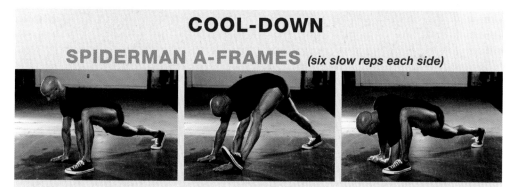

WARM-UP

Jumping Jacks (for sixty seconds)

Then do eight reps of each of these exercises, for two rounds total:

SIDE-LYING LEG LIFTS   ITB LEG LIFTS   BACKSTROKE

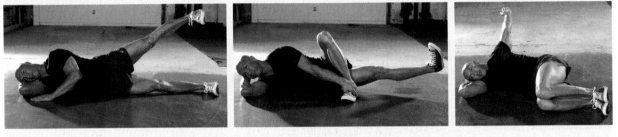

WORKOUT

40/20 WORK-TO-REST INTERVALS.

Y CUFF

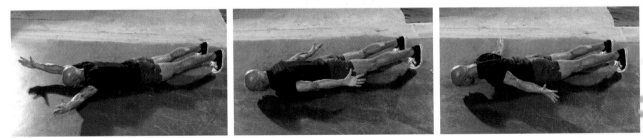

HIGH KICK

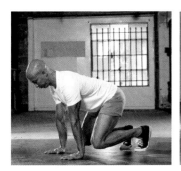 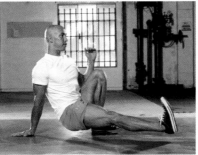 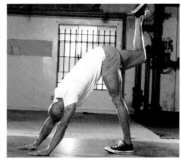

HIGH-KNEE RUN

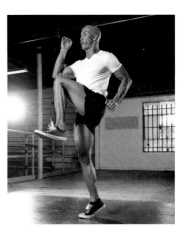

Shin muscles, glutes, hip flexors, hip rotators, hamstrings, quadriceps, calves, abs, obliques, spinal erectors, deltoids, lats, traps, hip abductors/adductors, biceps, neck

You're running in place. Stand up straight with your midsection tight, swing your arms, and get your knees up! Your elbows should remain bent at ninety degrees. Keep your knees and toes pointing straight ahead. Find a fast and relaxed pace that you can maintain for the entire work interval. You'll need to coordinate your breath with your legs. This is a tough one that's as hard as you're willing to make it. Think of it this way—the world record 400-meter dash is only 43.03 seconds!

COOL-DOWN

SPIDERMAN A-FRAMES *(six slow reps each side)*

WARM-UP

Jumping Jacks (for sixty seconds)

Then do eight reps of each of these exercises, for two rounds total:

SIDE-LYING LEG LIFTS   ITB LEG LIFTS   BACKSTROKE

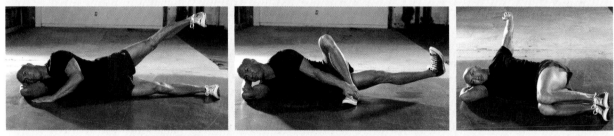

WORKOUT

40/20 WORK-TO-REST INTERVALS.

PARALLEL LEG BRIDGE

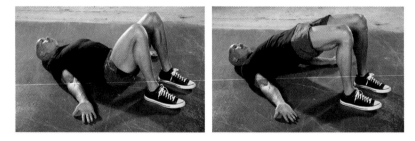

HIGH DROP

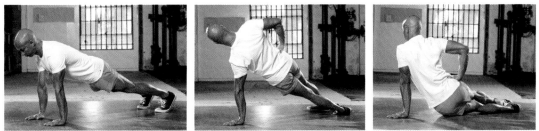

T-ARM SQUAT

TIPS: Fully extend through your arms, fingertips to fingertips. You should have a perfectly straight line between your hands. Proprioception, which is knowing where you are in space, is one of the most important skills we develop with exercise. You need it for everything, and it makes learning new skills so much easier. (In fact, did you know there's technically more than five senses? And proprioception is one of them!)

Fight for every millimeter of range of motion through all parts of your body. Don't be sloppy. Continuously scan your body by feel to make sure you're executing everything with perfect form.

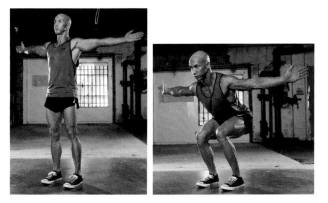

COOL-DOWN

SPIDERMAN A-FRAMES *(six slow reps each side)*

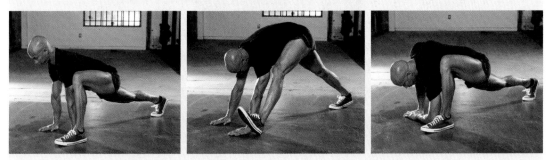

WARM-UP

March in Place (for sixty seconds)

Then do eight reps of each of these exercises, for two rounds total:

HIP CIRCLES TWIST AND REACH POINTERS

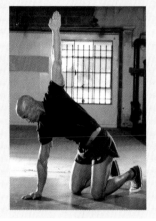
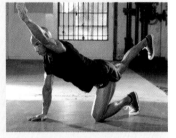

WORKOUT

40/20 WORK-TO-REST INTERVALS.

BENT LEG BRIDGE

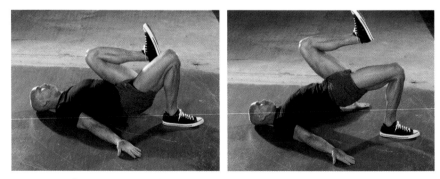

STARFISH DROP

Deltoids, pectorals, triceps, forearms, lats, spinal erectors, abs, obliques, rib muscles, hip flexors, glutes, shin muscles, calves, hamstrings, quadriceps, hip abductors/adductors, biceps, neck

This is just like the Starfish Twist except you're dropping all the way down to the bottom of a Push-Up in the middle of the movement. You then push yourself back up to the starting position of a Push-Up and switch sides.

If a perfect Push-Up is too hard, it's okay to "worm" yourself up. Focus on controlling the transitions down to the bottom of a Push-Up with a perfectly straight body position. You know the deal: Flex your glutes, lift your chest slightly, tighten your abs, and tuck your chin slightly. Similarly, make yourself straight in the side planking positions as well.

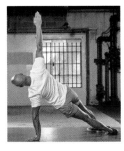 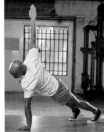 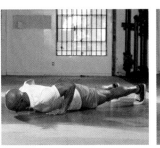 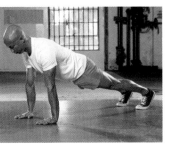

HIGH-KNEE MARCH

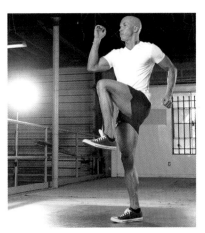

COOL-DOWN

SPIDERMAN ARM CIRCLES *(eight reps each side)*

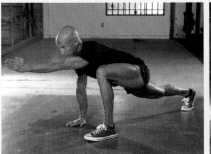 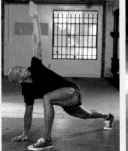 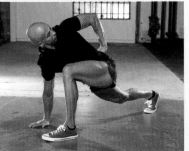

WARM-UP

March in Place (for sixty seconds)

Then do eight reps of each of these exercises, for two rounds total:

HIP CIRCLES   TWIST AND REACH   POINTERS

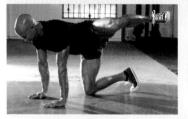
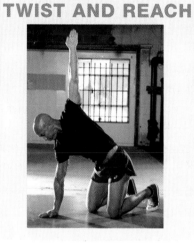
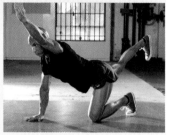

WORKOUT

40/20 WORK-TO-REST INTERVALS.

Y CUFF

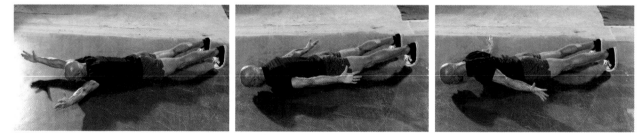

HIGH KICK

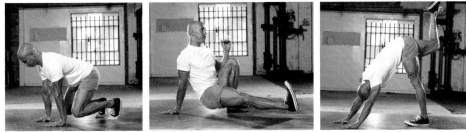

SQUAT THRUST

Shin muscles, glutes, hip rotators, hamstrings, quadriceps, calves, obliques, spinal erectors, deltoids, triceps, forearms, lats, abs, hip flexors, pectorals, biceps, neck

Get into a squatting position with your feet hip- to shoulder-width apart and parallel. Your knees should point straight ahead with your hips back and your chest up.

INHALE: Transition to the starting position of a Push-Up by placing your hands on the floor and kicking both feet back in one fluid movement. Make yourself long and straight from head to heels in the Push-Up position.

EXHALE: In one fluid movement, pop back up to the squatting position with your feet parallel, knees pointing straight ahead, hips back, and chest up.

The Squat should look and feel like an athletic ready position from which you could instantly jump, sprint, or catch a ball.

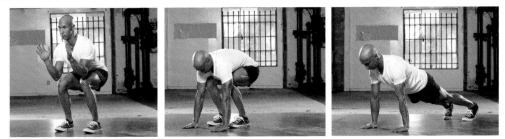

COOL-DOWN

SPIDERMAN ARM CIRCLES *(eight reps each side)*

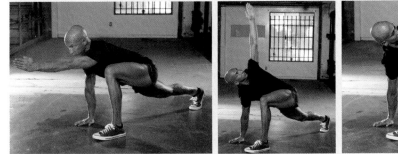
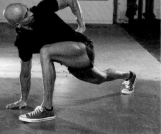

WARM-UP

March in Place (for sixty seconds)

Then do eight reps of each of these exercises, for two rounds total:

HIP CIRCLES　　TWIST AND REACH　　POINTERS

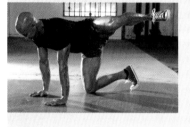
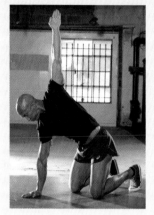
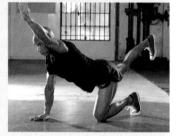

WORKOUT

40/20 WORK-TO-REST INTERVALS.

BENT LEG CRUNCH

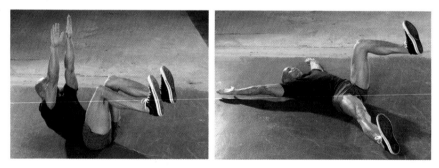

SIDE KICK

Deltoids, triceps, forearms, abs, hip flexors, obliques, spinal erectors, lats, calves, hamstrings, glutes, quadriceps, shin muscles, internal hip rotators, rib muscles, traps, neck

After doing a Kickout, get to the top of a High Kick position.

From there, reach the right foot up and over your left side, like a scorpion stinger, until you get a good stretch along the right side of your body. Make the supporting leg as straight as possible, and keep your chest pushed down toward the supporting foot.

Reset to starting position and switch sides. Exhale in the end positions: Kickouts and Side Kick.

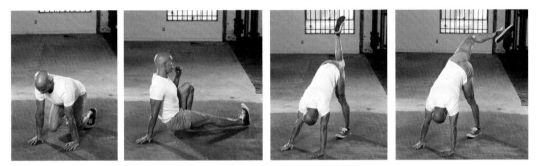

STORK STANCE

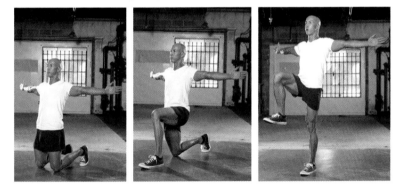

COOL-DOWN

SPIDERMAN ARM CIRCLES *(eight reps each side)*

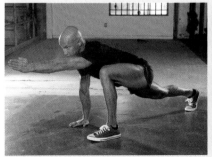
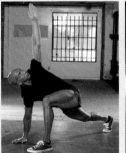
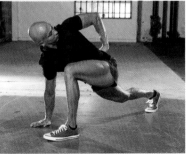

WARM-UP

March in Place (for sixty seconds)

Then do eight reps of each of these exercises, for two rounds total:

HIP CIRCLES   TWIST AND REACH   POINTERS

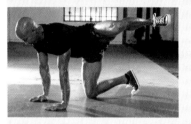
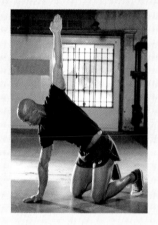
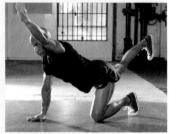

WORKOUT

40/20 WORK-TO-REST INTERVALS.

ARM HAULERS

TIP: Flex your glutes, suck in your belly button, keep your chest on the floor, and tuck your chin slightly.

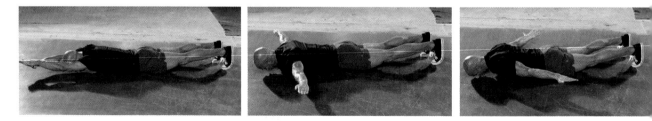

LOW DROP

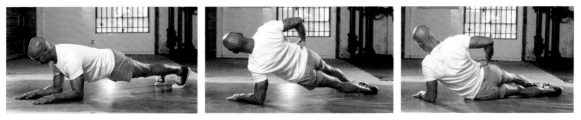

STREAMLINE DEAD LIFT

TIP: After each rep, make yourself tall. Flex your glutes, lift your chest slightly, and exhale fully.

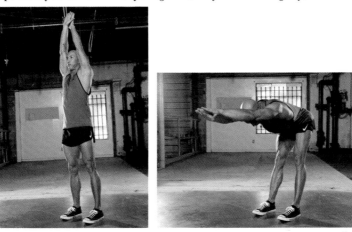

COOL-DOWN

SPIDERMAN ARM CIRCLES *(eight reps each side)*

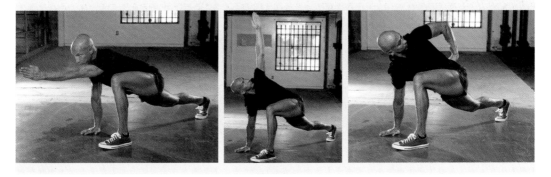

WARM-UP

Jumping Jacks (for sixty seconds)

Then do eight reps of each of these exercises, for two rounds total:

SIDE-LYING LEG LIFTS   ITB LEG LIFTS   BACKSTROKE

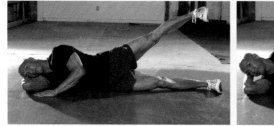 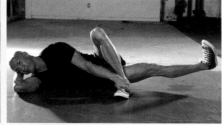 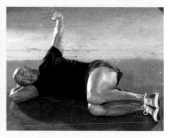

WORKOUT

45/15 WORK-TO-REST INTERVALS.

T-ARM REACH

Rear deltoids, rib muscles, shoulder rotators, traps, shin muscles, quadriceps, glutes, abs, spinal erectors, lats, neck, triceps, forearms

Get to a front lying position with both hands behind your back.

INHALE: Pull the left hand under your armpit and extend it to the T position so that it's perpendicular to your body, thumb up.
EXHALE: Raise the left thumb as high as you can.
INHALE: Lower your arm.
EXHALE: Pull your hand under your armpit, and return it on your lower back.

Switch sides.

Keep your pelvis pushed into the floor, navel drawn in, and chest on the floor as you raise your arms at the T position. Challenge your range of motion and ability to move your arms around a long and stable spine.

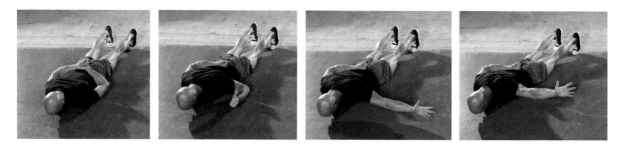

STARFISH DROP

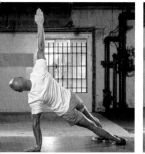 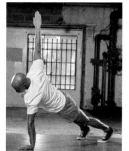 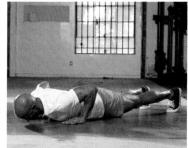 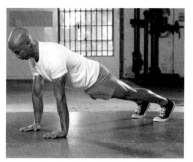

HIGH-KNEE RUN

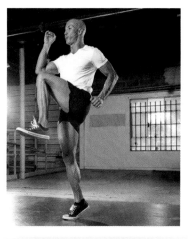

COOL-DOWN

BLOOMERS *(eight slow reps)*

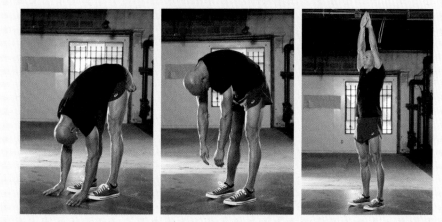

WARM-UP

Jumping Jacks (for sixty seconds)

Then do eight reps of each of these exercises, for two rounds total:

SIDE-LYING LEG LIFTS   ITB LEG LIFTS   BACKSTROKE

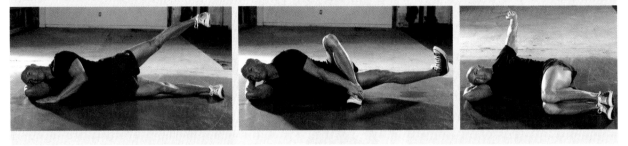

WORKOUT

45/15 WORK-TO-REST INTERVALS.

BENT LEG CRUNCH

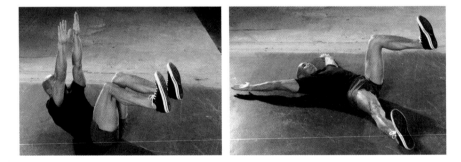

KICKOUT

TIP: After each Kickout, as you reset to the quadruped starting position, place your feet so that your knees remain close to your hands. This makes the exercise slightly easier while teaching you to pay attention to your footwork.

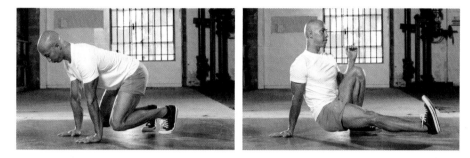

SQUAT THRUST

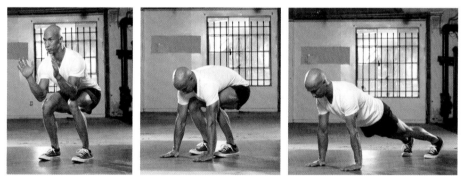

COOL-DOWN

BLOOMERS *(eight slow reps)*

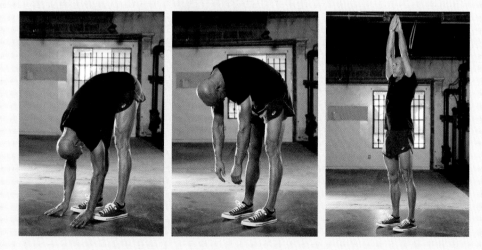

WARM-UP

Jumping Jacks (for sixty seconds)

Then do eight reps of each of these exercises, for two rounds total:

SIDE-LYING LEG LIFTS   ITB LEG LIFTS   BACKSTROKE

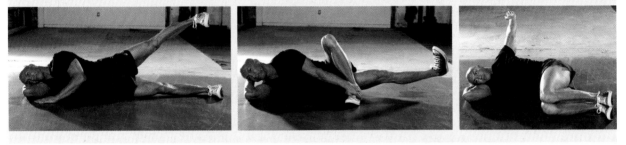

WORKOUT

45/15 WORK-TO-REST INTERVALS.

BENT LEG BRIDGE

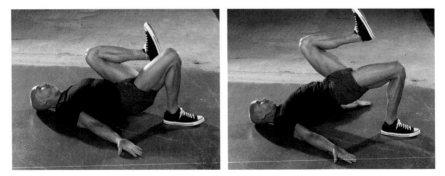

DOUBLE FUN GLIDE

Pectorals, deltoids, triceps, abs, hip flexors, hamstrings, calves, shin muscles, spinal erectors, lats, forearms, quadriceps, glutes, rib muscles, traps, neck

Get to the starting position of a Push-Up with your feet hip-width apart and your wrists directly under your shoulders.

Push your hips up into the air while pushing your chest down toward your feet. Let your heels sink down toward the floor. You should feel a good stretch in the back of your legs.

INHALE: Lower yourself to the bottom of a Push-Up.
EXHALE: Drive yourself back up to the starting position.

Think of this exercise as a Push-Up where you push your hips up into the air to get a good stretch after every rep.

To make this exercise easier, worm yourself up to the starting position of a Push-Up, and then get your hips up into the air. Focus on a controlled descent with a long, straight body position at the end.

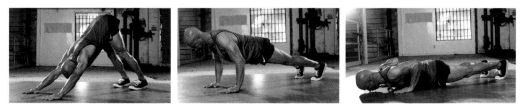

STREAMLINE ROMANIAN DEAD LIFT

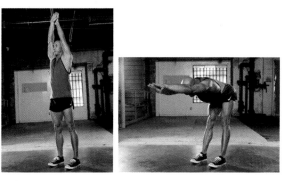

COOL-DOWN

BLOOMERS *(eight reps each side)*

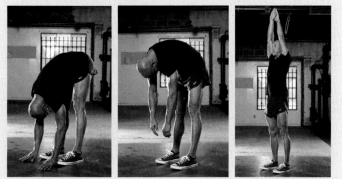

WARM-UP

Jumping Jacks (for sixty seconds)

Then do eight reps of each of these exercises, for two rounds total:

SIDE-LYING LEG LIFTS   ITB LEG LIFTS   BACKSTROKE

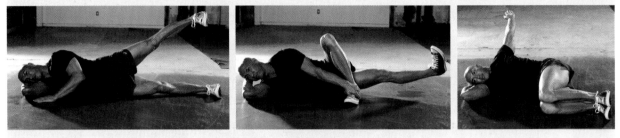

WORKOUT

45/15 WORK-TO-REST INTERVALS.

T-ARM REACH

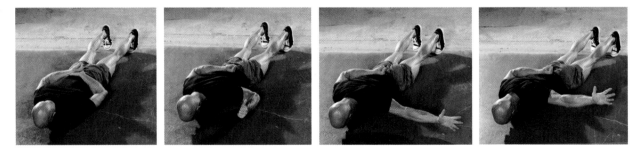

HIGH DROP

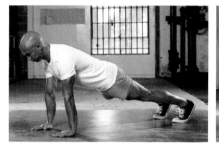
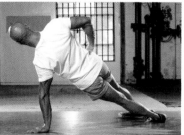
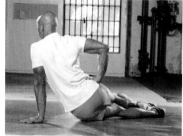

T-ARM SQUAT

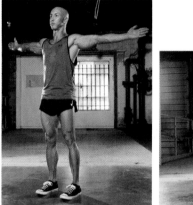
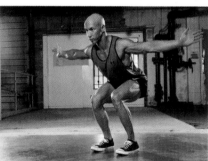

COOL-DOWN

BLOOMERS *(eight slow reps)*

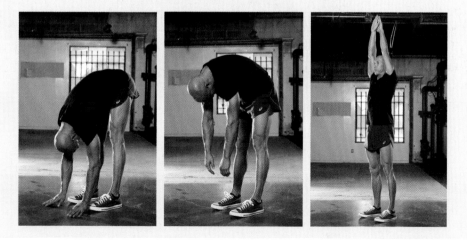

WARM-UP

March in Place (for sixty seconds)

Then do eight reps of each of these exercises, for two rounds total:

HIP CIRCLES   TWIST AND REACH   POINTERS

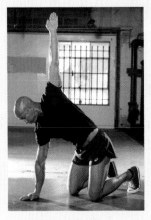
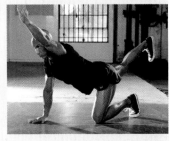

WORKOUT

45/15 WORK-TO-REST INTERVALS.

BENT LEG CRUNCH

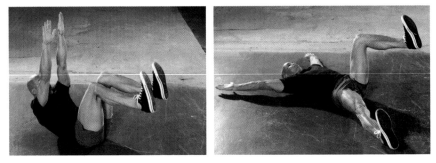

SIDE KICK

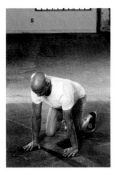 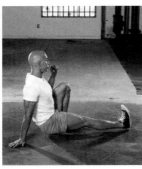 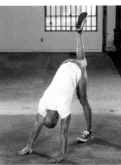 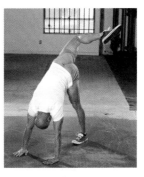

HIGH-KNEE SKIP

Shin muscles, glutes, hip flexors, hip rotators, hamstrings, quadriceps, calves, abs, obliques, spinal erectors, deltoids, lats, traps, hip abductors/adductors, biceps, neck

We're skipping in place. If you're one of those few who already know how to do it, wonderful. But for those of us who don't:

Begin by running in place, nice and easy. Keep your knees low for now.

After a few steps on each side, add one-second pauses to each step, so that you're briefly holding up each knee. Get the rhythm of that.

Next, add a small one-legged hop to each step. You should now be skipping in place!

As you improve, get your knees up higher, and use a stronger arm swing. If you absolutely can't get the High-Knee Skip down, use the High-Knee Run or High-Knee March instead.

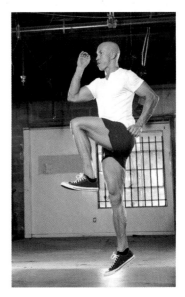

COOL-DOWN

STRADDLE REACH *(eight reps each side)*

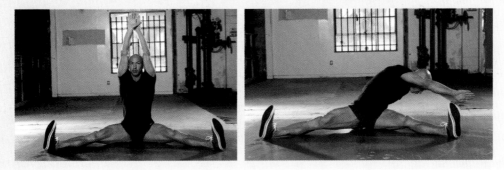

WARM-UP

March in Place (for sixty seconds)

Then do eight reps of each of these exercises, for two rounds total:

HIP CIRCLES

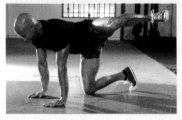

TWIST AND REACH

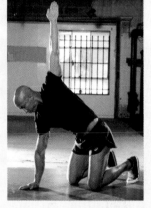

POINTERS

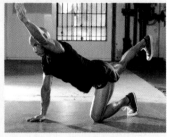

WORKOUT

45/15 WORK-TO-REST INTERVALS.

BENT LEG BRIDGE

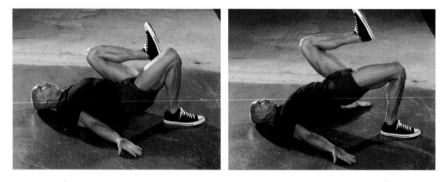

LOW DROP

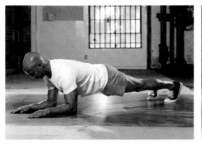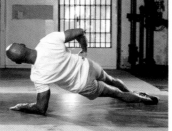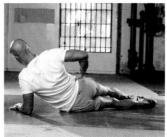

BOTTOM SQUAT

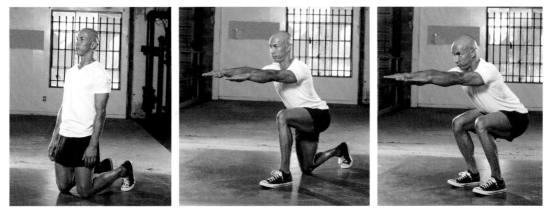

COOL-DOWN

STRADDLE REACH (eight reps each side)

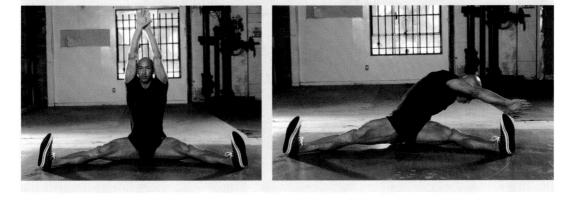

WARM-UP

March in Place (for sixty seconds)

Then do eight reps of each of these exercises, for two rounds total:

HIP CIRCLES   TWIST AND REACH   POINTERS

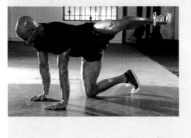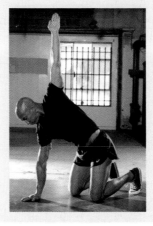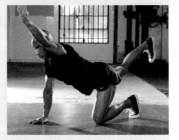

WORKOUT

45/15 WORK-TO-REST INTERVALS.

Y CUFF

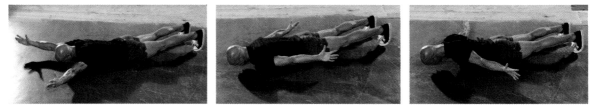

STARFISH DROP

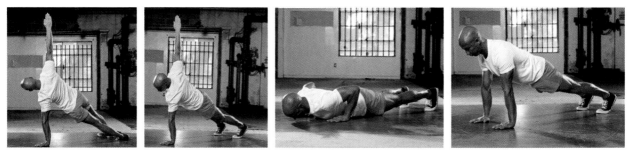

ROMANIAN DEAD LIFT TO SQUAT

Glutes, hamstrings, quadriceps, lats, traps, spinal erectors, shin muscles, deltoids, calves, abs, triceps, forearms, neck, hip rotators

Get into the starting position of a Streamline Romanian Dead Lift with your feet parallel and hip-width apart.

INHALE: With your legs straight, push your hips back and hip hinge forward until you feel a stretch in your hamstrings. Push your hips back and reach forward while keeping your legs as straight as possible.
EXHALE: Then transition to the bottom of a T-Arm Squat by bending your knees, dropping your hips, lifting your chest, and extending your arms fully to the T position.
INHALE: Return to the bottom of a Streamline Romanian Dead Lift by straightening your legs and reaching past your head.
EXHALE: Stand up tall and straight to complete the rep.

Make sure your feet stay parallel through every rep, and keep your knees pointing straight ahead.

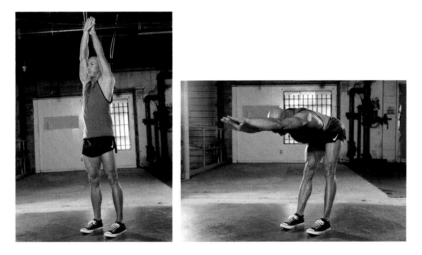

COOL-DOWN

STRADDLE REACH *(eight reps each side)*

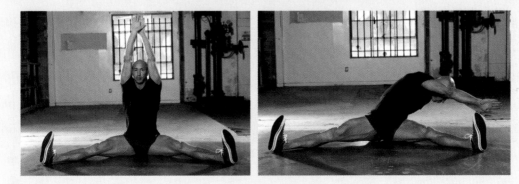

WARM-UP

March in Place (for sixty seconds)

Then do eight reps of each of these exercises, for two rounds total:

HIP CIRCLES　TWIST AND REACH　POINTERS

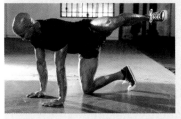
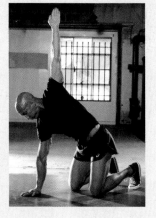
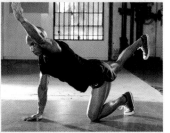

WORKOUT

45/15 WORK-TO-REST INTERVALS.

ARM HAULERS

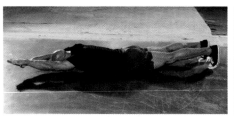
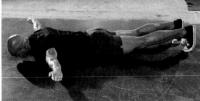
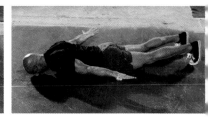

SIDE KICK

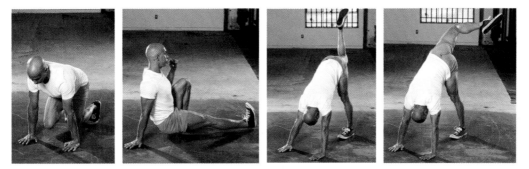

STORK STANCE

TIP: Get your knees up as high as you can while fully extending through the supporting leg so that you're as tall and straight as humanly possible. You should feel an awesome squeeze in your glute.

Also, pull the toes of the raised foot up, as if you're marching in place.

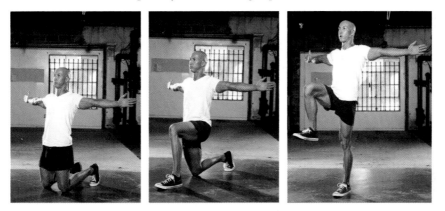

COOL-DOWN

STRADDLE REACH *(eight reps each side)*

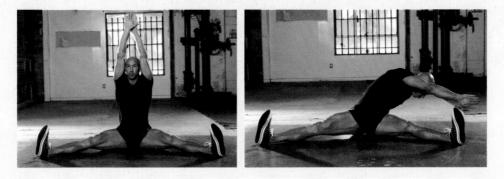

WARM-UP

Jumping Jacks (for sixty seconds)

Then do eight reps of each of these exercises, for two rounds total:

SIDE-LYING LEG LIFTS   ITB LEG LIFTS   BACKSTROKE

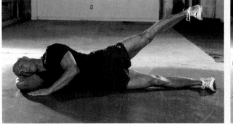 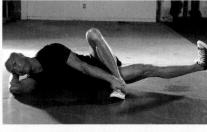 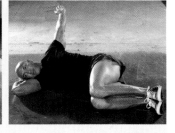

WORKOUT

50/10 WORK-TO-REST INTERVALS.

PARALLEL LEG BRIDGE

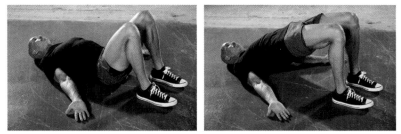

KICKOUT

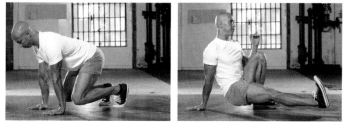

SIDE SQUAT

Shin muscles, glutes, hip rotators, hip abductors/adductors, hamstrings, quadriceps, calves, obliques, spinal erectors, hip flexors, abs, lats, deltoids, traps

Start in a tall double kneeling position.

INHALE: Take a big step forward with the left leg and get into a long single kneeling position with your arms held out front.

EXHALE: Shift your weight onto your left leg and rotate forty-five degrees to the right until your left leg is bent about ninety degrees and your right leg is straight.

INHALE: Reverse the movement back into a single kneeling position.

EXHALE: Transition from single kneeling to double kneeling.

Switch sides.

In the Side Squat position, rotate until your feet are parallel and your bent knee is pointing in the same direction as your toes. Keep your hips low and get your chest up!

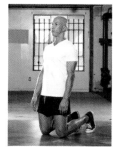
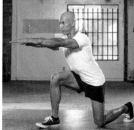
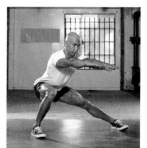
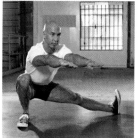

COOL-DOWN

ISOMETRIC
PIGEON STRETCH

(8 x 10 seconds on each side)

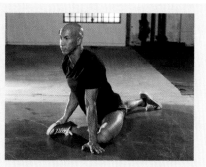

WARM-UP

Jumping Jacks (for sixty seconds)

Then do eight reps of each of these exercises, for two rounds total:

SIDE-LYING LEG LIFTS   ITB LEG LIFTS   BACKSTROKE

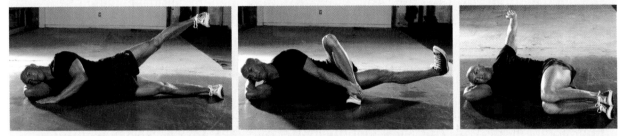

WORKOUT

50/10 WORK-TO-REST INTERVALS

T-ARM REACH

TIP: Coordinate your movements with your breathing.

Inhale as you extend your arm to the T position. Exhale *forcefully* as you raise your arm. Inhale as you lower it. Exhale as you set your arm on your lower back again. Switch sides.

Syncing your movements with your breath is the fastest and easiest way to improve coordination, performance, and strength. You can feel the difference instantly.

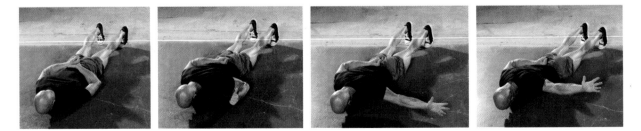

HIGH KICK

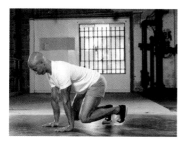 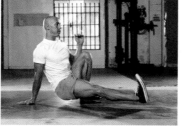 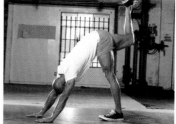

SQUAT THRUST

After every rep, focus on getting your chest up in the squatting position while exhaling.

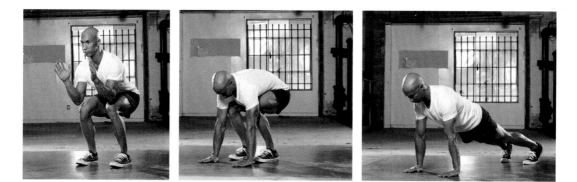

COOL-DOWN
ISOMETRIC PIGEON STRETCH
(8 x 10 seconds on each side)

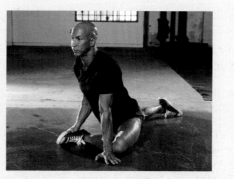

WARM-UP

Jumping Jacks (for sixty seconds)

Then do eight reps of each of these exercises, for two rounds total:

SIDE-LYING LEG LIFTS   ITB LEG LIFTS   BACKSTROKE

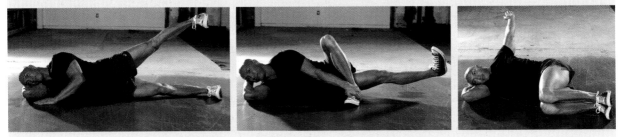

WORKOUT

50/10 WORK-TO-REST INTERVALS.

BENT LEG CRUNCH

TIPS: Challenge your range of motion!

At the bottom of the movement, while keeping your lower back in contact with the floor, reach past your head as far as possible, and blow out all your air.

Also, fully straighten your legs as you bring them down and to the side with your knees and toes turned straight up to the sky.

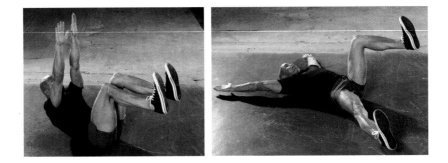

DOUBLE FUN GLIDE

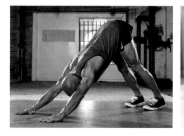 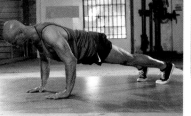 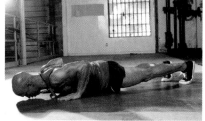

HIGH-KNEE SKIP

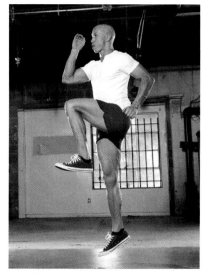

COOL-DOWN

ISOMETRIC
PIGEON STRETCH
(8 x 10 seconds on each side)

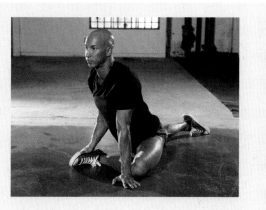

WARM-UP

Jumping Jacks (for sixty seconds)

Then do eight reps of each of these exercises, for two rounds total:

SIDE-LYING LEG LIFTS   ITB LEG LIFTS   BACKSTROKE

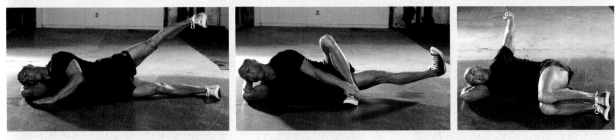

WORKOUT

50/10 WORK-TO-REST INTERVALS.

Y CUFF

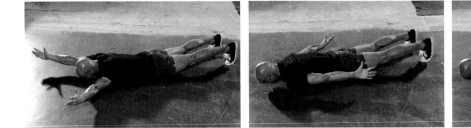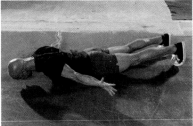

DOUBLE DROP

Deltoids, triceps, forearms, lats, spinal erectors, abs, obliques, rib muscles, hip flexors, glutes, shin muscles, calves, hamstrings, quadriceps, hip abductors/adductors, pectorals, biceps, neck

This is just like the High Drop, except that you're doing two reps before switching sides.

From the starting position of a Push-Up, roll your heels all the way left. Transition to a side planking position on your left side with your right arm on your hips.

INHALE: Lower your hips to the floor.
EXHALE: Raise your hips and make yourself perfectly straight head to heels.

Repeat and then switch sides.

After each hip drop, push your hips forward slightly, lift your chest, tighten your abs, and get your head in line with the rest of your body. Don't look at yourself as you do this exercise.

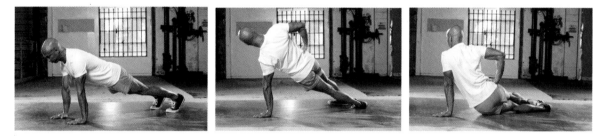

SIDE SQUAT

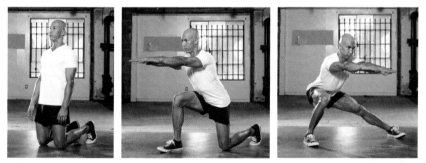

COOL-DOWN

ISOMETRIC
PIGEON STRETCH

(8 x 10 seconds on each side)

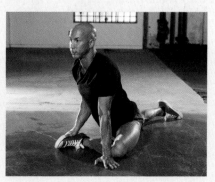

WARM-UP

March in Place (for sixty seconds)

Then do eight reps of each of these exercises, for two rounds total:

HIP CIRCLES   TWIST AND REACH   POINTERS

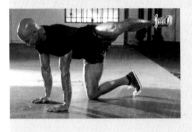
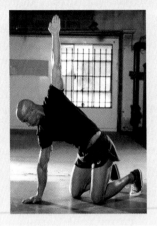
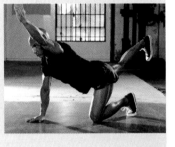

WORKOUT

50/10 WORK-TO-REST INTERVALS.

ARM HAULERS

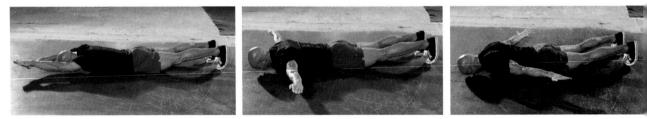

SIDE KICK

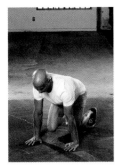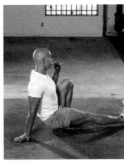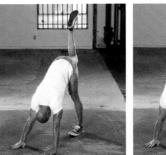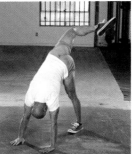

DROP THRUST

Shin muscles, glutes, hip rotators, hamstrings, quadriceps, calves, obliques, spinal erectors, deltoids, triceps, forearms, lats, abs, hip flexors, pectorals, biceps, neck

Similar to a Squat Thrust, but you progress here to adding in a dynamic Push-Up motion.

Get into an athletic ready position with your feet parallel and hip-to shoulder-width apart. Your knees should point straight ahead, with your hips back, and your chest up.

INHALE: In one fluid motion, place your hands on the floor, kick your feet back, and sink directly into the bottom of a Push-Up with your body lying on the floor, hands underneath your shoulders.
EXHALE: Pop back up to a standing position with your feet parallel, knees pointing straight ahead, hips back, and chest up.

Focus on transitioning in and out of a good squatting position.

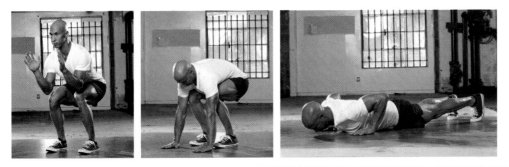

COOL-DOWN

HIP ROLLS *(eight slow reps)*

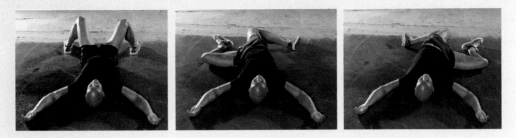

WARM-UP

March in Place (for sixty seconds)

Then do eight reps of each of these exercises, for two rounds total:

HIP CIRCLES   TWIST AND REACH   POINTERS

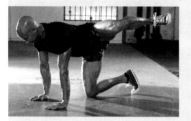
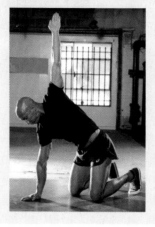
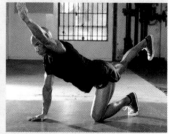

WORKOUT

50/10 WORK-TO-REST INTERVALS.

BENT LEG CRUNCH

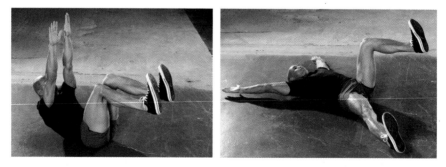

STARFISH TWIST

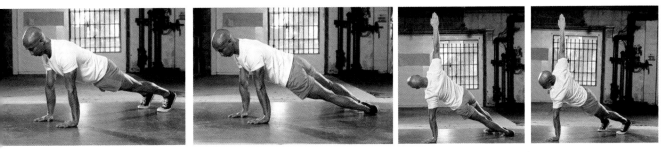

ROMANIAN DEAD LIFT TO SQUAT

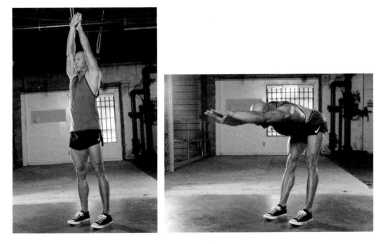

COOL-DOWN

HIP ROLLS *(eight slow reps)*

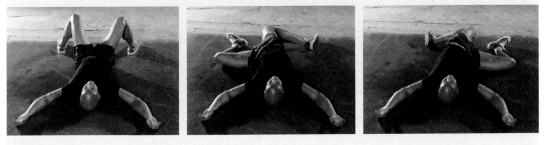

WARM-UP

March in Place (for sixty seconds)

Then do eight reps of each of these exercises, for two rounds total:

HIP CIRCLES   TWIST AND REACH   POINTERS

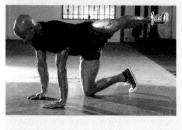
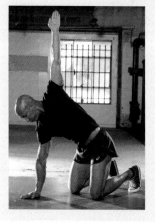
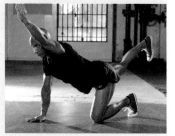

WORKOUT

50/10 WORK-TO-REST INTERVALS.

STRAIGHT LEG BRIDGE

Glutes, hamstrings, hip flexors, abs, shin muscles, quadriceps, spinal erectors, lats, lower/mid traps, deltoids, forearms

Get into the starting position of a Bent Leg Bridge with your right knee pulled to your chest. Straighten the right leg and press your right heel straight up to the sky. Keep the elevated ankle dorsiflexed with the toes pulled down toward your face. Pretend you're balancing a cup of tea on your foot.

EXHALE: Raise your hips as high as you can, and flex your abs at the top.
INHALE: Lower your hips.

Repeat for two reps, then switch legs.

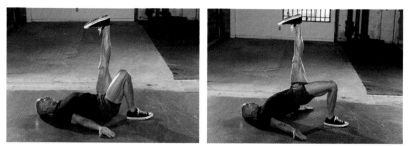

DOUBLE DROP

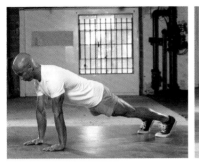 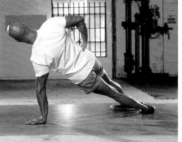 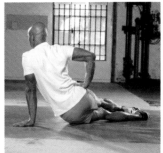

SIDE SQUAT

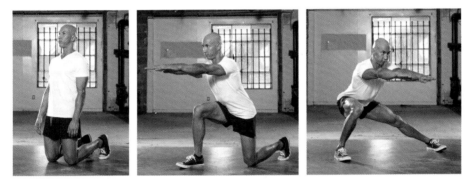

COOL-DOWN

HIP ROLLS *(eight slow reps)*

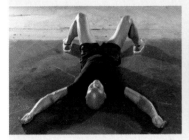 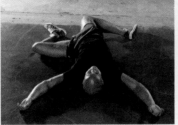 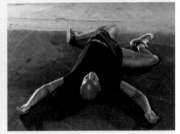

WARM-UP

March in Place (for sixty seconds)

Then do eight reps of each of these exercises, for two rounds total:

HIP CIRCLES TWIST AND REACH POINTERS

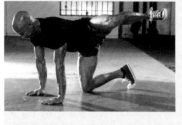
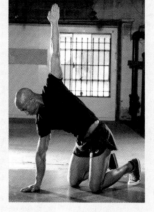
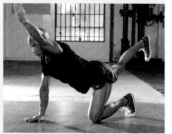

WORKOUT

50/10 WORK-TO-REST INTERVALS.

T-ARM REACH

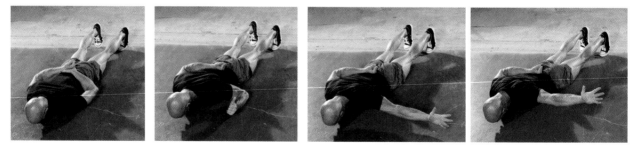

KICKOUT

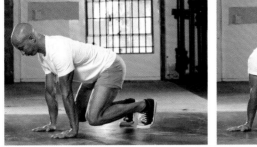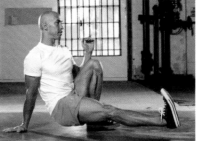

DROP THRUST

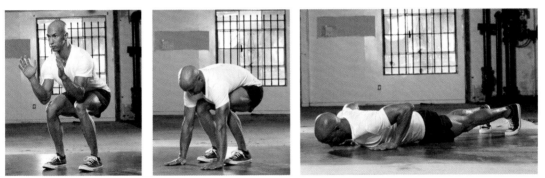

COOL-DOWN

HIP ROLLS *(eight slow reps)*

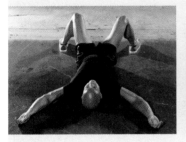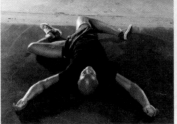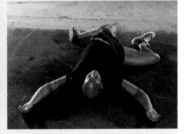

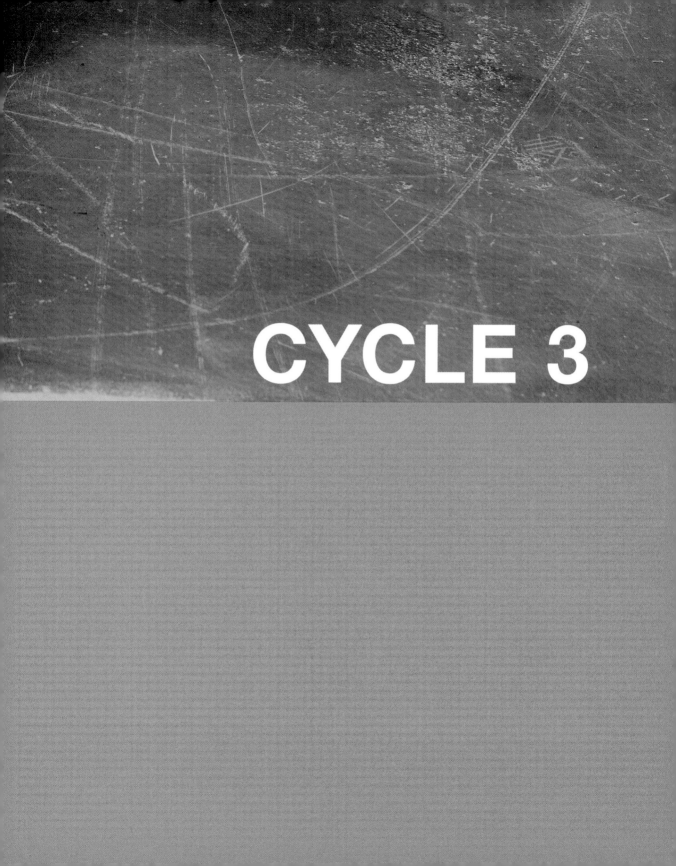

CYCLE 3

Strong and Lean *has proven to build more muscle than weight lifting, burn more fat than cardio, and produce sexier and safer results than either of those. It will turn your body into the only fitness equipment you'll ever need again.*

WARM-UP

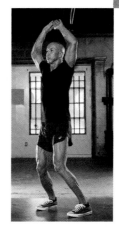

Jumping Jacks (for sixty seconds)

Then do eight reps of each of these exercises, for two rounds total:

SIDE-LYING LEG LIFTS

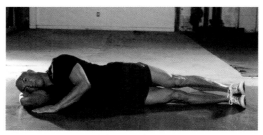

ITB LEG LIFTS

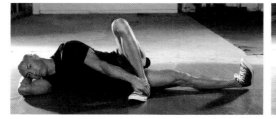
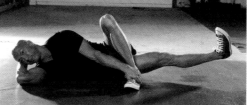

BACKSTROKE

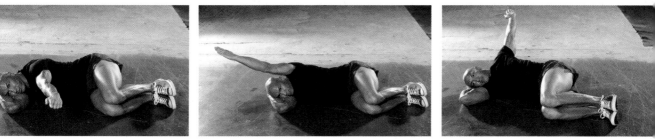

DOUBLE FUN GLIDE

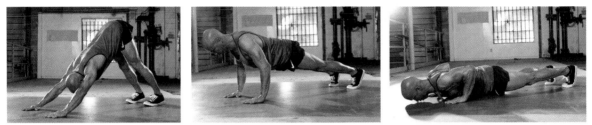

LET ME INS

Lats, rear deltoids, traps, biceps, forearms, glutes, hamstrings, spinal erectors, quadriceps, shin muscles, abs, obliques, neck

Grab some suspension straps* that are anchored to the top of a doorway or any overhead anchor point as shown, and pull the handles to your chest with your feet forward of the handles. Stand tall with the handles pulled to your chest. You should have a slight backward lean.

INHALE: Sink into a Squat and fully straighten your arms. Get a stretch between your shoulder blades at the bottom of the exercise.
EXHALE: Reset to a tall standing position and pull the handles into your chest again. At the top, squeeze your shoulder blades together and pull the handles apart.

You can make the exercise harder by moving your feet forward so that you have more of a backward lean.

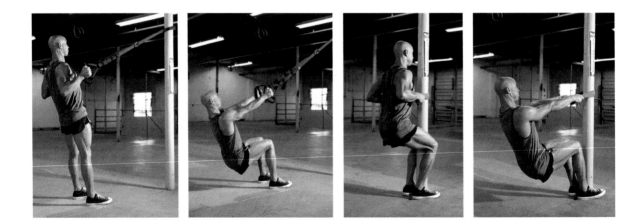

---

* If you don't have suspension straps, you can wrap a small hand towel around the handles of a sturdy door. Wrapping a rope or towel around a sturdy pole or railing also works great, as shown. If you use these variations, keep your hips and knees bent at ninety degrees throughout this exercise.

ROMANIAN DEAD LIFT TO SQUAT

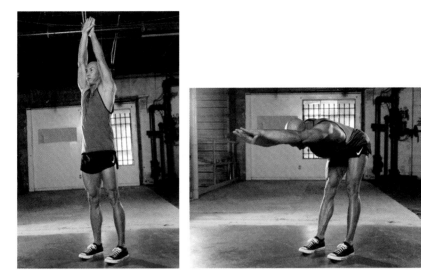

COOL-DOWN

SPIDERMAN A-FRAMES *(eight slow reps each side)*

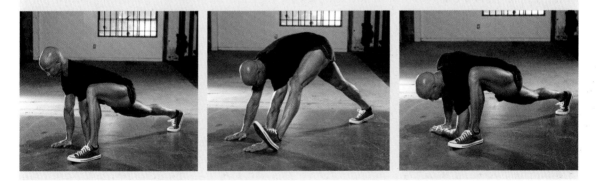

WARM-UP

Jumping Jacks (for sixty seconds)

Then do eight reps of each of these exercises, for two rounds total:

SIDE-LYING LEG LIFTS   ITB LEG LIFTS   BACKSTROKE

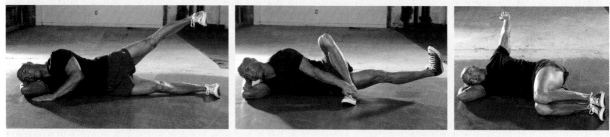

WORKOUT

50/10 WORK-TO-REST INTERVALS.

STRAIGHT LEG BRIDGE

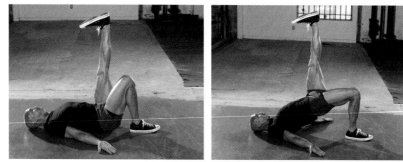

SIDE KICK

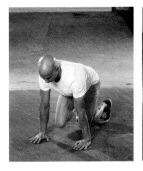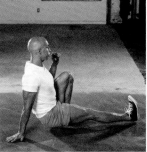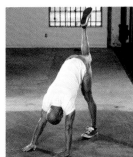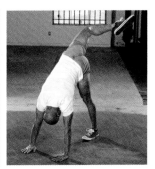

STORK STANCE

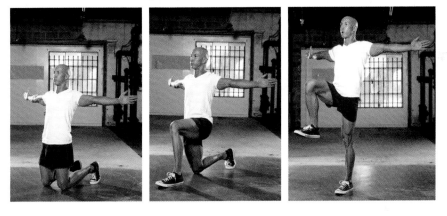

COOL-DOWN

SPIDERMAN ARM CIRCLES *(eight reps each side)*

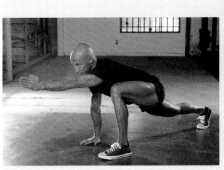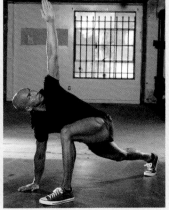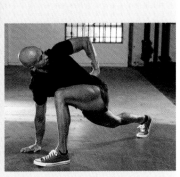

WARM-UP

Jumping Jacks (for sixty seconds)

Then do eight reps of each of these exercises, for two rounds total:

SIDE-LYING LEG LIFTS   ITB LEG LIFTS   BACKSTROKE

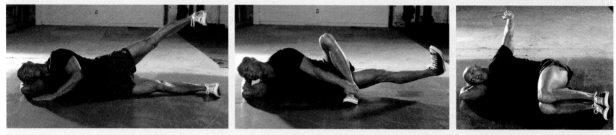

WORKOUT

50/10 WORK-TO-REST INTERVALS.

STRAIGHT LEG CRUNCH

Abs, hip flexors, obliques, neck, deltoids, shin muscles, quadriceps, glutes, hip rotators, rib muscles, traps

This is just like the Bent Leg Crunch except you're keeping both legs straight, or at least as straight as possible. Dorsiflex both ankles by pulling your toes down toward your face, and keep your feet parallel. To get into the starting position, reach up past your feet.

EXHALE: Lower your arms past your head to the Y position while keeping your lower back flat on the floor. At the same time, lower your left leg down and to the left side, while keeping the knee and toes of your left leg pointing straight up.

INHALE: Return to the starting position and switch legs for the next rep.

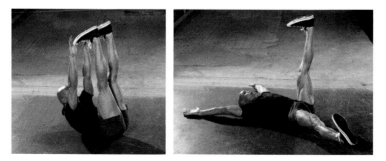

STARFISH DROP

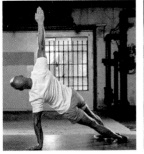 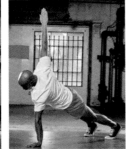 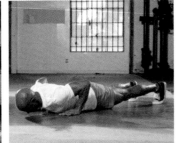 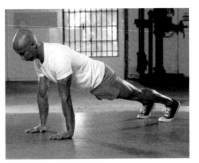

T-ARM SQUAT

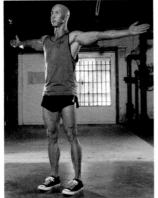 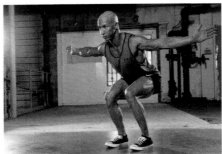

COOL-DOWN

BLOOMERS *(eight slow reps)*

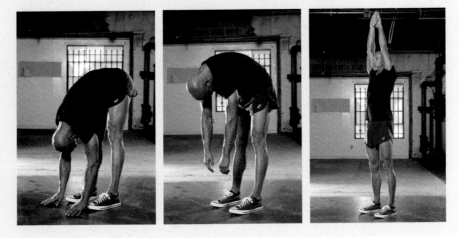

WARM-UP

Jumping Jacks (for sixty seconds)

Then do eight reps of each of these exercises, for two rounds total:

SIDE-LYING LEG LIFTS   ITB LEG LIFTS   BACKSTROKE

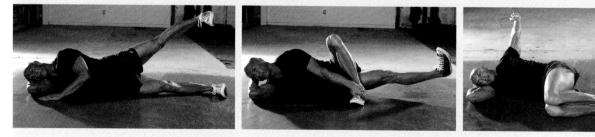

WORKOUT

50/10 WORK-TO-REST INTERVALS.

T-ARM REACH

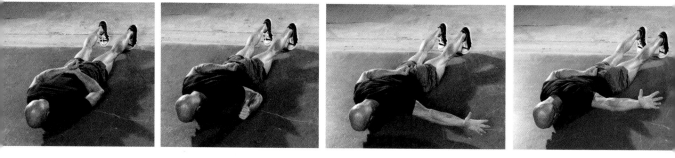

KICKOUT

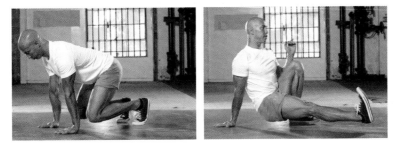

SIDE SQUAT

TIPS: Remember, keep your hips low and chest up as you transition from single kneeling to Side Squat. Get your feet parallel with the bent knee pointing in the same direction as your toes.

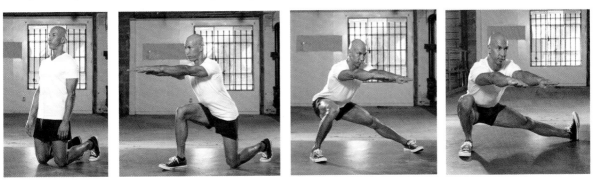

COOL-DOWN

STRADDLE REACH *(eight reps each side)*

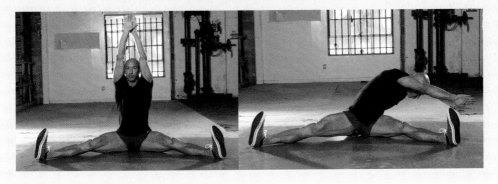

SIDE-LYING WARM-UP

Jumping Jacks (for sixty seconds)

Then do eight reps of each of these exercises, for two rounds total:

SIDE-LYING LEG LIFTS   ITB LEG LIFTS   BACKSTROKE

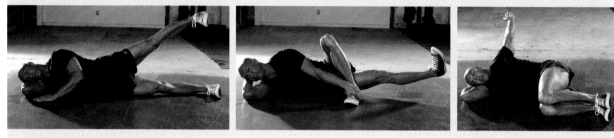

WORKOUT

40/20 WORK-TO-REST INTERVALS.

LOW DROP

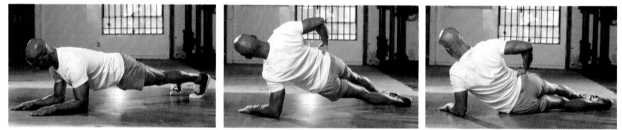

LET ME UPS

Lats, rear deltoids, traps, biceps, forearms, glutes, hamstrings, spinal erectors, quadriceps, shin muscles, abs, obliques, neck

You need something about hip height that you can lie underneath to pull yourself up with, such as suspension straps or a sturdy desk or table.

Lie on your back with your feet pulled in toward your hips so that your knees are bent. Reach up and grab whatever you're using to pull yourself up on. Raise your hips and make yourself perfectly straight from head to knees by tightening both your glutes and abs.

EXHALE: Pull your chest up between your hands, and squeeze your shoulder blades together at the top.
INHALE: Lower yourself to the starting position and fully straighten your arms to complete the rep.

Keep yourself as straight as possible throughout this exercise by getting your hips up and tightening your abs.

If this exercise is too hard, you can use Let Me Ins. Conversely, you can put your feet up on a chair or anything sturdy and knee height to make it more difficult.

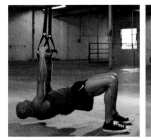 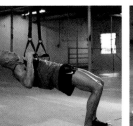 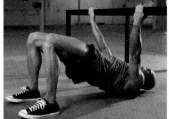 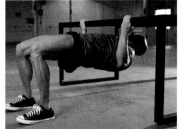

DROP THRUST

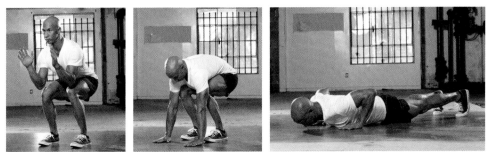

COOL-DOWN

ISOMETRIC PIGEON STRETCH
(8 x 10 seconds on each side)

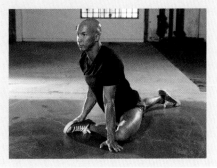

WARM-UP

March in Place (for sixty seconds)

Then do eight reps of each of these exercises, for two rounds total:

HIP CIRCLES   TWIST AND REACH   POINTERS

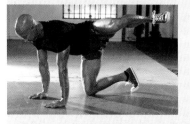
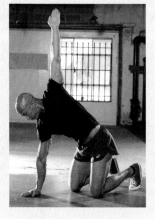
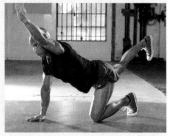

WORKOUT

50/10 WORK-TO-REST INTERVALS.

BENT LEG CRUNCH

TIP: Reach up high, exhale on the way down, and keep your lower back in contact with the floor at the bottom.

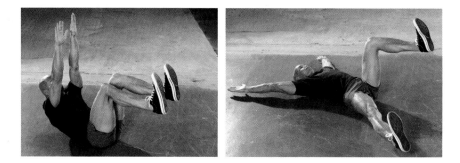

HIGH KICK

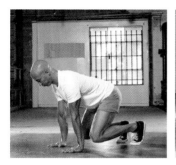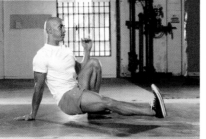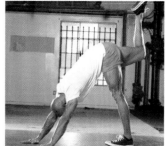

SQUAT THRUST

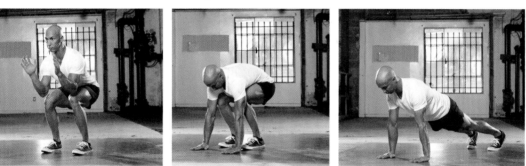

COOL-DOWN

HIP ROLLS *(eight slow reps)*

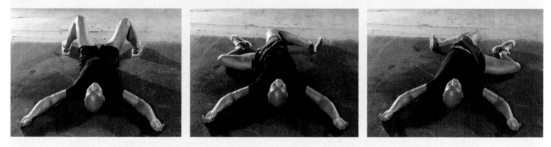

WARM-UP

March in Place (for sixty seconds)

Then do eight reps of each of these exercises, for two rounds total:

HIP CIRCLES   TWIST AND REACH   POINTERS

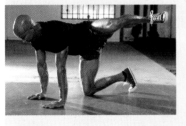
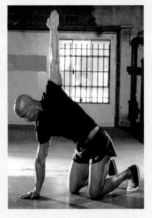
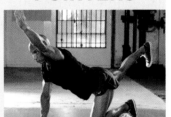

WORKOUT

50/10 WORK-TO-REST INTERVALS.

STRAIGHT LEG BRIDGE

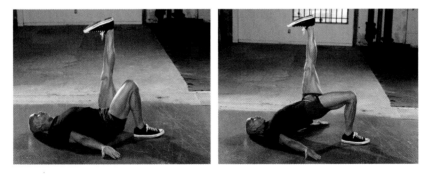

T-ARM REACH

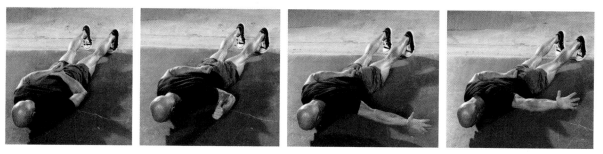

STORK STANCE

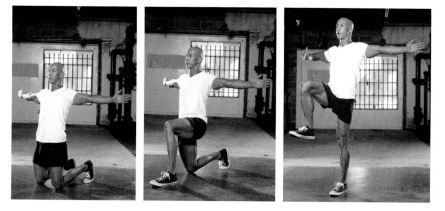

COOL-DOWN

SPIDERMAN A-FRAMES *(eight slow reps each side)*

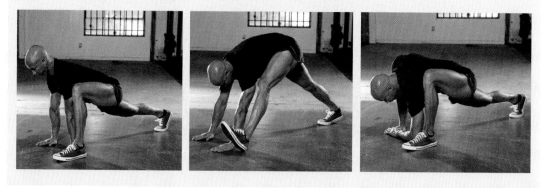

WARM-UP

March in Place (for sixty seconds)

Then do eight reps of each of these exercises, for two rounds total:

HIP CIRCLES   TWIST AND REACH   POINTERS

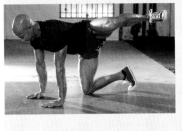
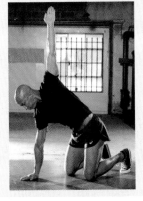
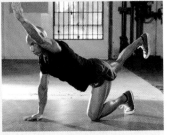

WORKOUT

40/20 WORK-TO-REST INTERVALS.

DOUBLE FUN GLIDE

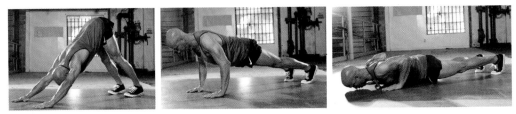

LET ME INS

TIP: Really squeeze your shoulder blades together at the top, and pull the handles apart as if you're Superman ripping his shirt off to expose the *S* on his chest.

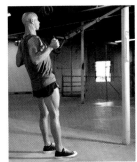
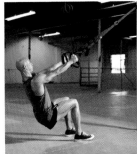
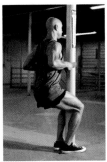
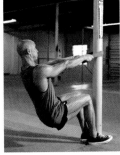

SQUAT TO ROMANIAN DEAD LIFT

Glutes, hamstrings, quadriceps, lats, traps, spinal erectors, shin muscles, deltoids, calves, abs, triceps, forearms, neck, hip rotators

This is the reverse of the Romanian Dead Lift to Squat. Get into the starting position for a T-Arm Squat.

INHALE: Push your hips back and down, and get into the bottom of a T-Arm Squat.

EXHALE: Straighten your legs and reach past your head in the bottom of a Streamline Romanian Dead Lift.

INHALE: Get back into the bottom of a T-Arm Squat by bending your knees, lifting your chest, and pulling your arms to the T position.

EXHALE: Stand up tall and straight to complete the rep.

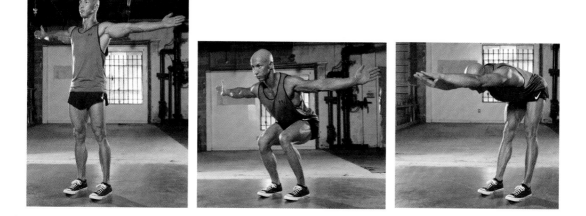

COOL-DOWN

SPIDERMAN ARM CIRCLES *(eight reps each side)*

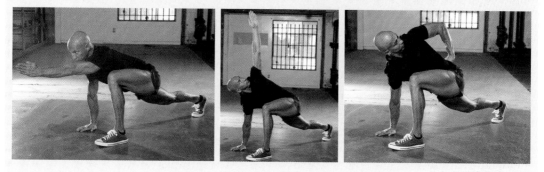

WARM-UP

March in Place (for sixty seconds)

Then do eight reps of each of these exercises, for two rounds total:

HIP CIRCLES   TWIST AND REACH   POINTERS

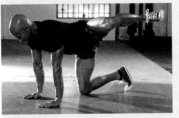
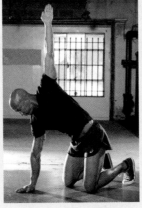
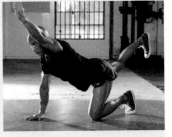

WORKOUT

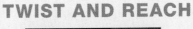

50/10 WORK-TO-REST INTERVALS.

ARM HAULERS

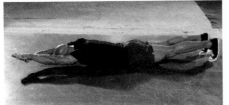
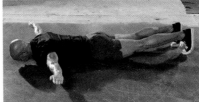
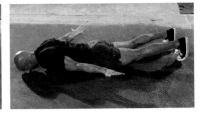

DOUBLE DROP

TIP: Remember, in the side planking positions, push your hips forward slightly, lift your chest, and get your head in position to make yourself perfectly straight.

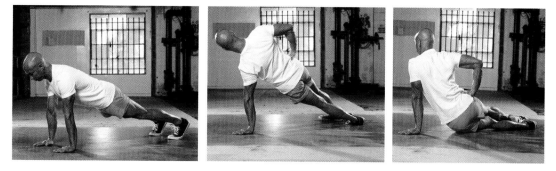

PARALLEL LEG BRIDGE

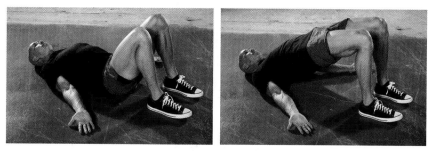

COOL-DOWN

BLOOMERS *(eight slow reps)*

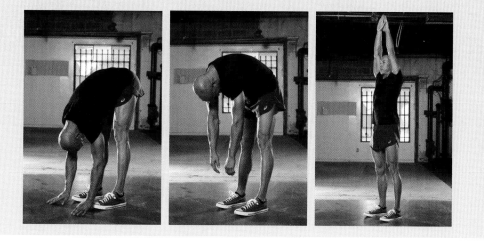

WARM-UP

March in Place (for sixty seconds)

Then do eight reps of each of these exercises, for two rounds total:

HIP CIRCLES   TWIST AND REACH   POINTERS

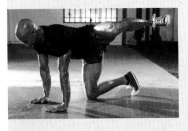
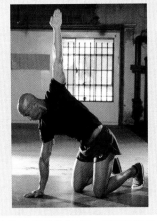
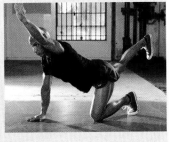

WORKOUT

50/10 WORK-TO-REST INTERVALS.

Y CUFF

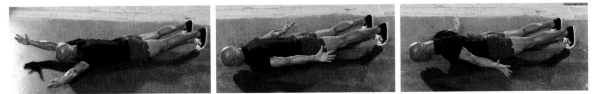

STARFISH TWIST

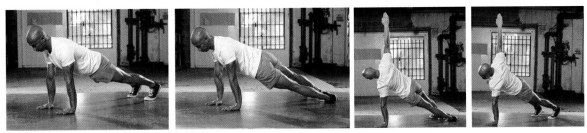

COSSACK SQUAT

Hamstrings, glutes, quadriceps, hip rotators, hip flexors, spinal erectors, obliques, calves, shin muscles, deltoids, traps, abs, lats

This move is a progression from the Side Squat. Get into a tall double kneeling position.

INHALE: Step forward with the left leg and get into a long single kneeling position with your arms raised to the front.

EXHALE: Rotate to the right and get into the Side Squat position. But let your hips sink down as far as possible while keeping your left foot flat on the floor. Lift your chest, and fully straighten the right leg while turning the toes and knee of the right leg up toward the sky.

INHALE: Return to a single kneeling position with your left leg forward.

EXHALE: Get to a tall double kneeling position.

Switch sides.

Don't rush. Exhale fully in the end positions. Let your hips sink and lift your chest.

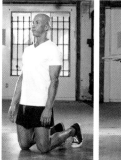 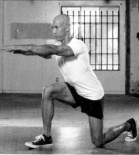 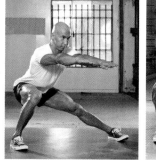 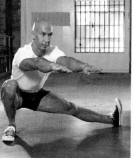

COOL-DOWN

STRADDLE REACH *(eight reps each side)*

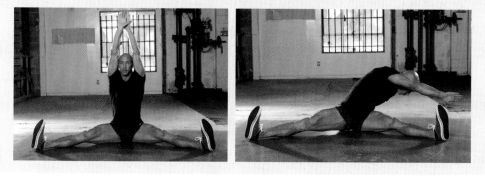

WARM-UP

Jumping Jacks (for sixty seconds)

Then do eight reps of each of these exercises, for two rounds total:

SIDE-LYING LEG LIFTS   ITB LEG LIFTS   BACKSTROKE

WORKOUT

45/15 WORK-TO-REST INTERVALS.

STARFISH BOUNCE

Deltoids, pectorals, triceps, forearms, lats, spinal erectors, abs, obliques, rib muscles, hip flexors, glutes, shin muscles, calves, hamstrings, quadriceps, hip abductors/adductors, biceps, neck

Do a Starfish Push-Up, but as soon as you get to the bottom of the Push-Up, drive yourself up as hard and fast as you can. Try to get some air! Catch yourself by immediately sinking into the bottom of another Push-Up. Reset to the top of the Push-Up, and switch sides.

If you can't get air, do two regular Push-Ups instead. Then switch sides.

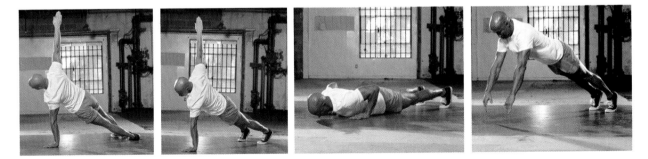

LET ME UPS

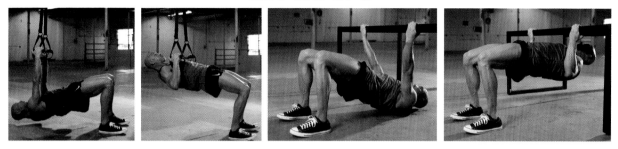

SQUAT TO ROMANIAN DEAD LIFT

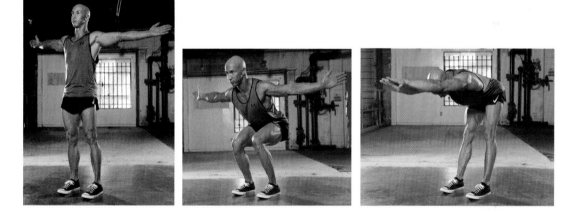

COOL-DOWN

ISOMETRIC PIGEON STRETCH
(8 x 10 seconds on each side)

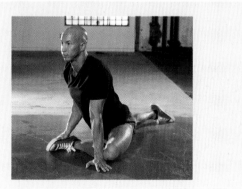

WARM-UP

Jumping Jacks (for sixty seconds)

Then do eight reps of each of these exercises, for two rounds total:

SIDE-LYING LEG LIFTS   ITB LEG LIFTS   BACKSTROKE

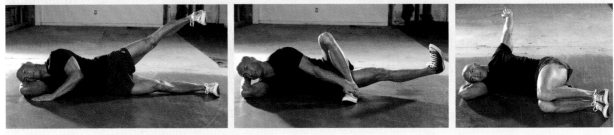

WORKOUT

50/10 WORK-TO-REST INTERVALS.

BENT LEG BRIDGE

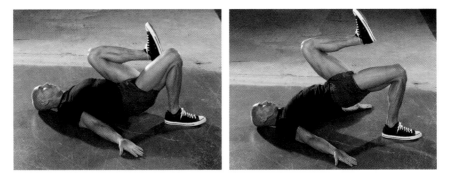

STORK STANCE

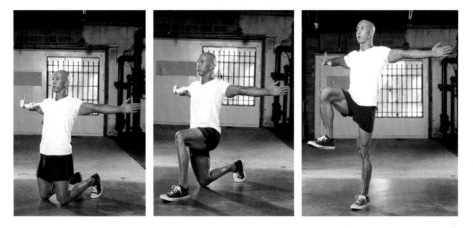

HIGH-KNEE RUN

TIPS: Focus on your posture by lifting your chest slightly while keeping your midsection tight. Make yourself tall and straight with a slight forward lean. Aggressively swing your arms and get your knees up.

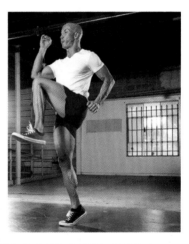

COOL-DOWN

HIP ROLLS *(eight slow reps)*

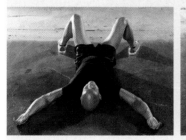
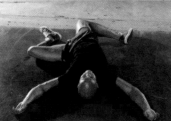
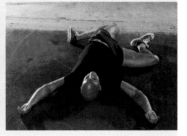

WARM-UP

Jumping Jacks (for sixty seconds)

Then do eight reps of each of these exercises, for two rounds total:

SIDE-LYING LEG LIFTS   ITB LEG LIFTS   BACKSTROKE

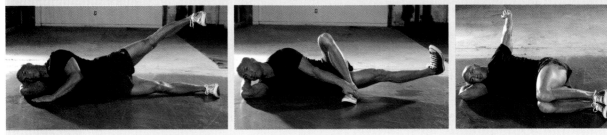

WORKOUT

50/10 WORK-TO-REST INTERVALS.

ARM HAULERS

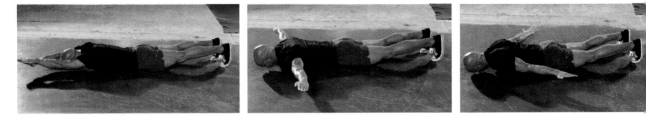

HIGH KICK

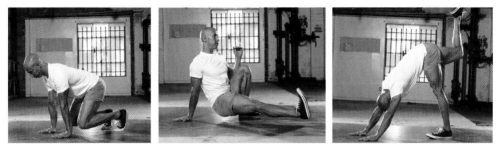

ROMANIAN DEAD LIFT TO SQUAT

TIPS: Remember, keep your feet parallel and knees pointing straight ahead. Get your hips down and chest up as you transition into the T-Arm Squat.

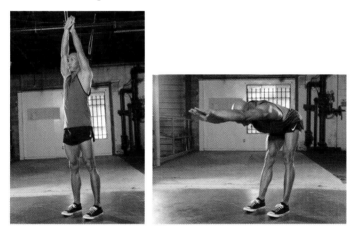

COOL-DOWN

SPIDERMAN A-FRAMES *(eight slow reps each side)*

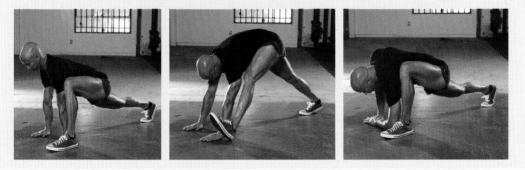

WARM-UP

Jumping Jacks (for sixty seconds)

Then do eight reps of each of these exercises, for two rounds total:

SIDE-LYING LEG LIFTS   ITB LEG LIFTS   BACKSTROKE

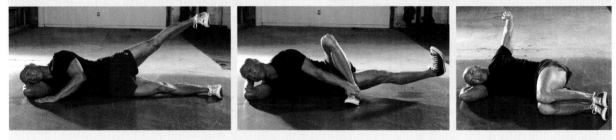

WORKOUT

50/10 WORK-TO-REST INTERVALS.

STRAIGHT LEG CRUNCH

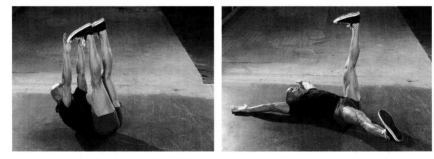

DOUBLE DROP

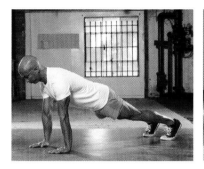 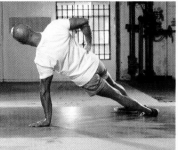 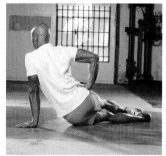

HIGH-KNEE SKIP

TIPS: As you lower one leg, you should already be pulling the other leg up. In other words, don't wait until the raised foot is on the floor before pulling up the other foot. Just like with the High-Knee Run, you should never have both feet on the floor at the same time.

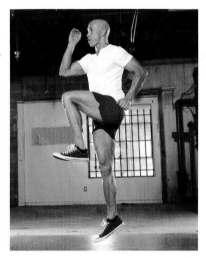

COOL-DOWN

SPIDERMAN ARM CIRCLES *(eight reps each side)*

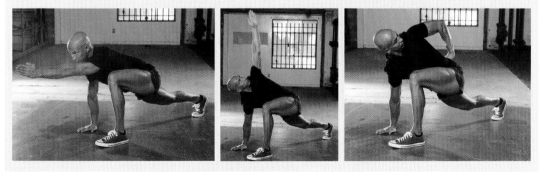

WARM-UP

Jumping Jacks (for sixty seconds)

Then do eight reps of each of these exercises, for two rounds total:

SIDE-LYING LEG LIFTS   ITB LEG LIFTS   BACKSTROKE

WORKOUT

45/15 WORK-TO-REST INTERVALS.

TRIPOD PRESS

Pectorals, deltoids, triceps, abs, obliques, hip flexors, hip rotators, hip abductors, shin muscles, glutes, hamstrings, calves, quadriceps, spinal erectors, lats, forearms, rib muscles, traps, neck

Get into a Push-Up position with your hands and feet shoulder-width apart.

Tense your glutes and tighten your midsection. Raise your left leg off the floor, and keep the knee and toes of the elevated leg pointing straight down.

INHALE: Lower yourself to the floor while keeping your body straight.
EXHALE: Drive yourself back up.

Do two reps with the left leg elevated, and then do two reps with the right leg elevated.

This exercise gets harder the wider your feet are apart. If you hit muscle failure, worm yourself back up to the starting position and focus on controlling the way down with a straight body position.

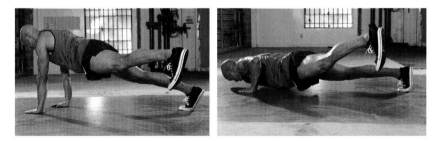

LET ME INS

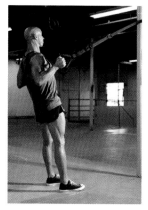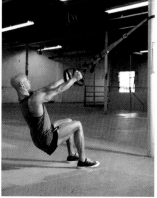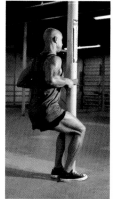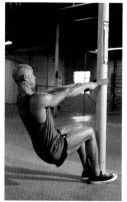

COSSACK SQUAT

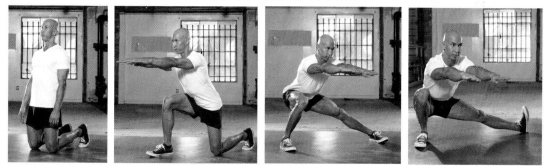

COOL-DOWN

BLOOMERS *(eight slow reps)*

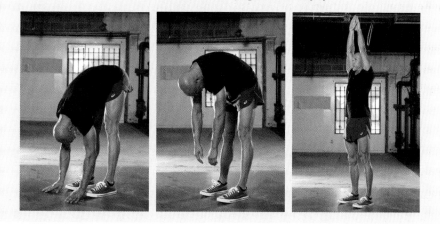

WARM-UP

March in Place (for sixty seconds)

Then do eight reps of each of these exercises, for two rounds total:

HIP CIRCLES   TWIST AND REACH   POINTERS

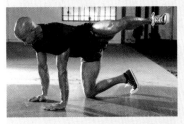
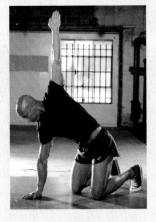
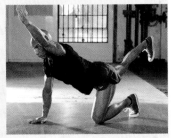

WORKOUT

50/10 WORK-TO-REST INTERVALS.

STRAIGHT LEG BRIDGE

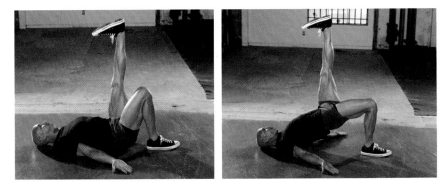

SIDE KICK

TIPS: Focus on getting a good Kickout and High Kick before transitioning to Side Kick. Exhale in the Kickout and Side Kick positions.

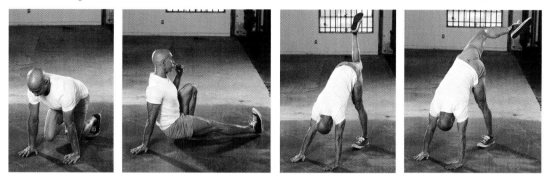

SQUAT THRUST

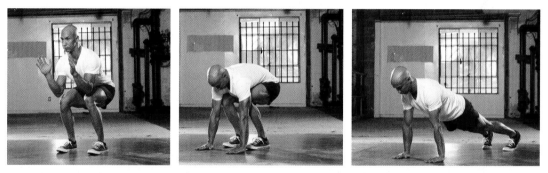

COOL-DOWN

STRADDLE REACH *(eight reps each side)*

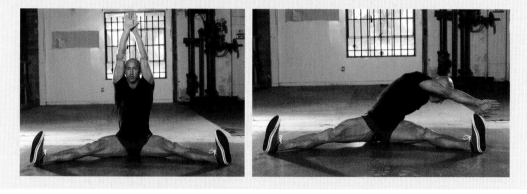

WARM-UP

March in Place (for sixty seconds)

Then do eight reps of each of these exercises, for two rounds total:

HIP CIRCLES   TWIST AND REACH   POINTERS

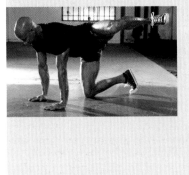
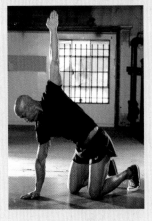
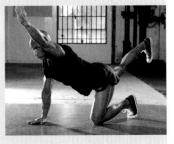

WORKOUT

50/10 WORK-TO-REST INTERVALS.

BENT LEG CRUNCH

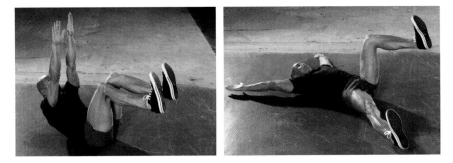

HIGH DROP

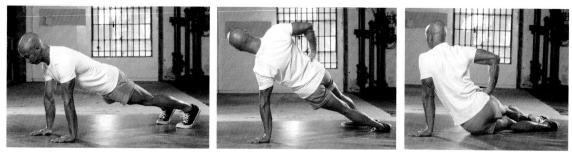

STORK STANCE

TIPS: Remember, in Stork Stance, fully straighten the supporting leg, squeeze your glutes, lift your chest, and tighten your abs to make yourself tall and straight. Fully extend through your arms and make them straight from fingertips to fingertips.

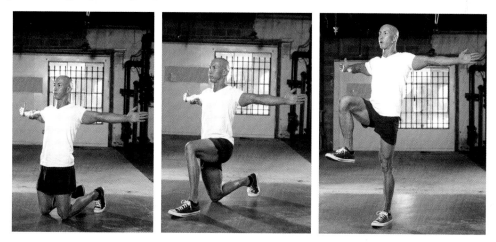

COOL-DOWN
ISOMETRIC
PIGEON STRETCH
(8 x 10 seconds on each side)

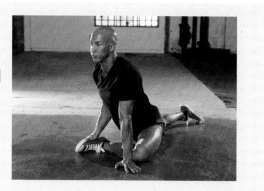

WARM-UP

March in Place (for sixty seconds)

Then do eight reps of each of these exercises, for two rounds total:

HIP CIRCLES   TWIST AND REACH   POINTERS

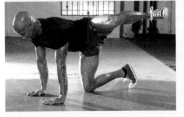
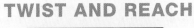
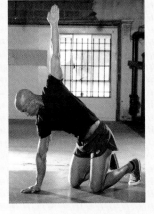
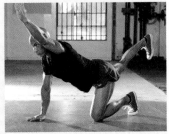

WORKOUT

45/15 WORK-TO-REST INTERVALS.

DOUBLE FUN GLIDE

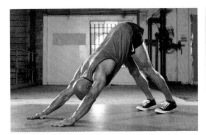
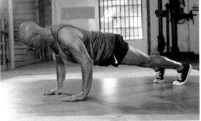
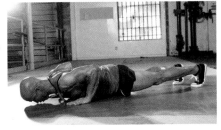

TRIPOD LET ME UPS

Lats, rear deltoids, traps, biceps, forearms, glutes, hamstrings, spinal erectors, quadriceps, shin muscles, hip rotators, hip abductors/adductors, abs, obliques, neck

Get into the starting position of Let Me Ups. Place your feet shoulder-width apart. Fully extend the left leg with the knee and toes of the left foot pointing straight up. Keep your hips level, meaning do not let your hips rotate down toward the side of the elevated leg. Keep a perfectly long and straight body position as you would for regular Let Me Ups. The wider your legs, the harder the exercise.

EXHALE: Pull yourself up as high as you can while keeping your body straight.
INHALE: Lower yourself until your arms are straight and you feel a light stretch between your shoulder blades.

Perform two reps, and then switch legs.

If Tripod Let Me Ups are too hard or become too hard during a set, put both feet down and switch to regular Let Me Ups. It's okay to do partial reps where you focus on making yourself straight in the bottom position and pulling yourself up as high as you can, even if it's just a few inches.

If you can't do Tripod Let Me Ups and Let Me Ups are not an option, use Let Me Ins.

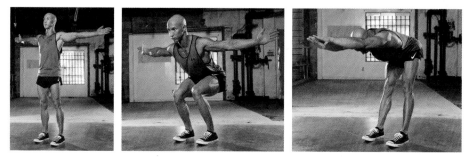

SQUAT TO ROMANIAN DEAD LIFT

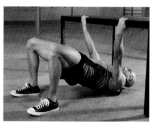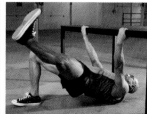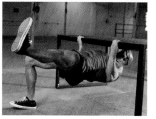

COOL-DOWN

HIP ROLLS *(eight slow reps)*

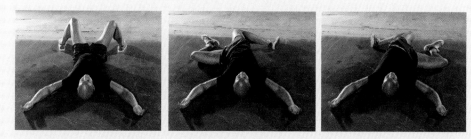

WARM-UP

March in Place (for sixty seconds)

Then do eight reps of each of these exercises, for two rounds total:

HIP CIRCLES   TWIST AND REACH   POINTERS

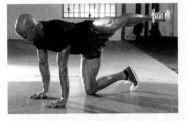
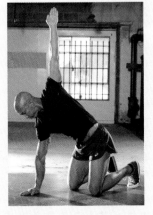
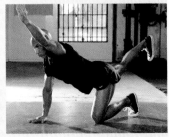

WORKOUT

50/10 WORK-TO-REST INTERVALS.

Y CUFF

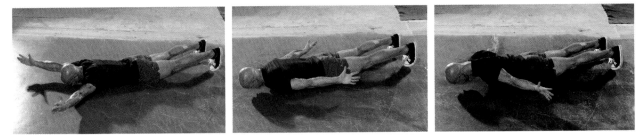

LOW DROP

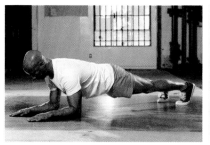
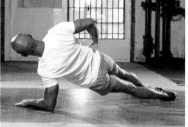
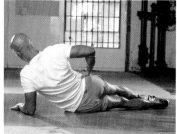

BOTTOM SQUAT

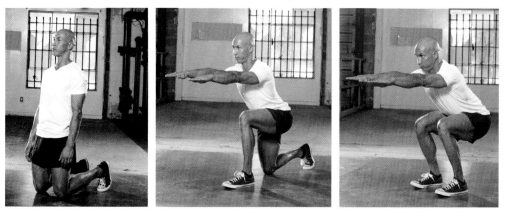

COOL-DOWN

SPIDERMAN A-FRAMES *(eight slow reps each side)*

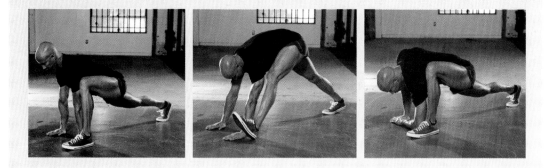

WARM-UP

March in Place (for sixty seconds)

Then do eight reps of each of these exercises, for two rounds total:

HIP CIRCLES   TWIST AND REACH   POINTERS

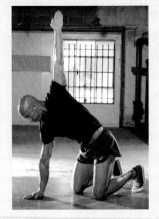

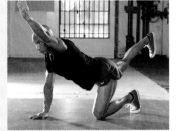

WORKOUT

50/10 WORK-TO-REST INTERVALS.

PARALLEL LEG BRIDGE

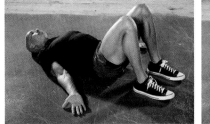

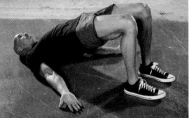

T-ARM REACH

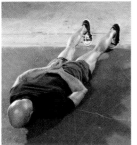
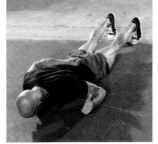
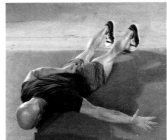
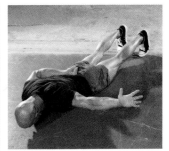

COSSACK SQUAT

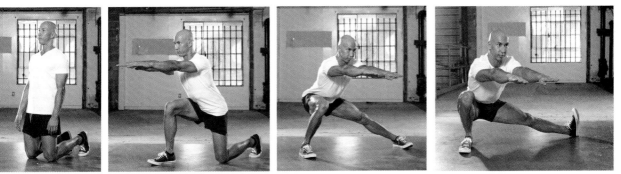

COOL-DOWN

SPIDERMAN ARM CIRCLES *(eight reps each side)*

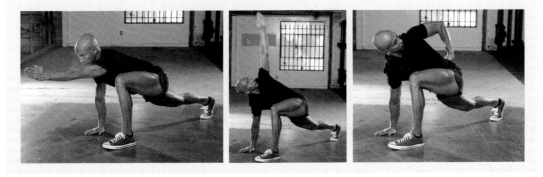

WARM-UP

Jumping Jacks (for sixty seconds)

Then do eight reps of each of these exercises, for two rounds total:

SIDE-LYING LEG LIFTS   ITB LEG LIFTS   BACKSTROKE

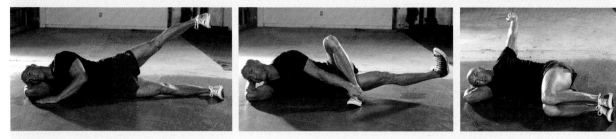

WORKOUT

50/10 WORK-TO-REST INTERVALS.

STARFISH BOUNCE

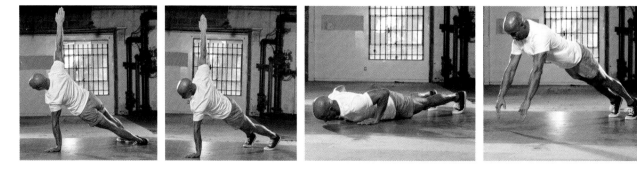

LET ME INS

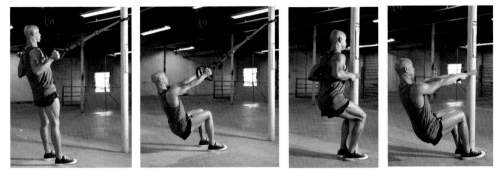

JUMP THRUST

Shin muscles, glutes, hip rotators, hamstrings, quadriceps, calves, obliques, spinal erectors, deltoids, triceps, forearms, lats, abs, hip flexors, pectorals, biceps, neck

Do a Squat Thrust, and then jump into the air using an arm swing. Try to land with your feet parallel and immediately push your hips back! Get right back into a good squatting position with your feet parallel, knees pointing straight ahead, hips back, and chest up.

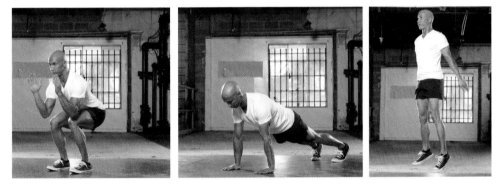

COOL-DOWN

BLOOMERS *(eight slow reps)*

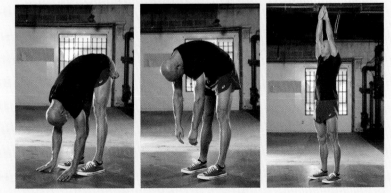

WARM-UP

Jumping Jacks (for sixty seconds)

Then do eight reps of each of these exercises, for two rounds total:

SIDE-LYING LEG LIFTS   ITB LEG LIFTS   BACKSTROKE

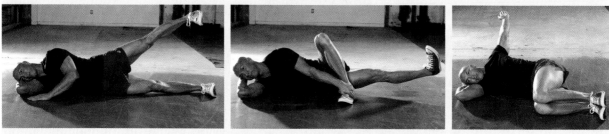

WORKOUT

50/10 WORK-TO-REST INTERVALS.

T-ARM REACH

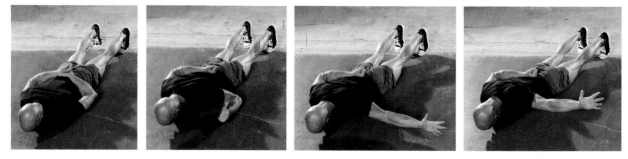

STRAIGHT LEG BRIDGE

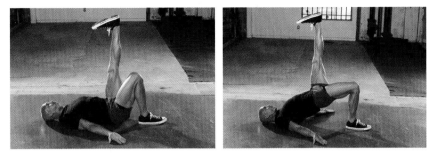

ROMANIAN DEAD LIFT TO SQUAT

TIP: Remember, for the Romanian Dead Lift portion of this exercise, fully straighten your legs.

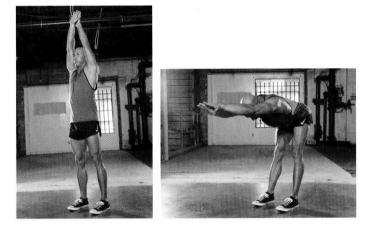

COOL-DOWN

STRADDLE REACH *(eight reps each side)*

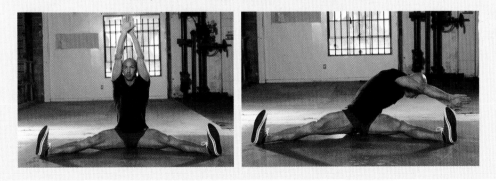

WARM-UP

Jumping Jacks (for sixty seconds)

Then do eight reps of each of these exercises, for two rounds total:

SIDE-LYING LEG LIFTS   ITB LEG LIFTS   BACKSTROKE

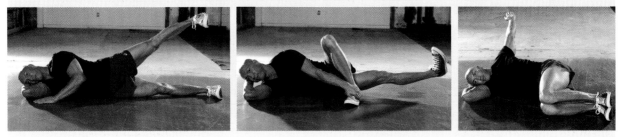

WORKOUT

50/10 WORK-TO-REST INTERVALS.

Y CUFF

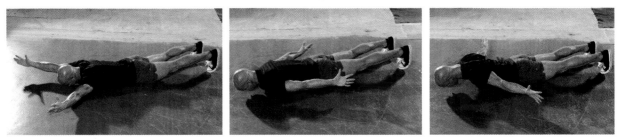

DIVE BOMBER

Deltoids, triceps, pectorals, abs, hip flexors, traps, hamstrings, calves, shin muscles, spinal erectors, lats, forearms, quadriceps, glutes, rib muscles, neck

Get into the starting position of a Push-Up with your feet hip-width apart and your hands shoulder-width apart. Push your hips up into the air, and push your chest down toward your feet.

INHALE: In a swooping dive bomber motion, lower your head between your arms and continue forward until your chest is between your hands. Then straighten your arms until your chest is up and you're facing forward.

EXHALE: Reverse the swooping motion by lowering your chest and raising your hips so that your chest is between your hands again. Then push your hips back up to the starting position.

TIPS: To make the exercise easier, raise your hips up directly from the bottom position without reversing the swooping downward motion. To make the exercise still easier, take out the swooping downward motion, and simply lower your hips straight down from the top position, and then raise them directly back up from the bottom position.

Take the time to get a good stretch in each end position. At the top, push your chest down toward your feet and straighten your legs. Let your heels sink down. At the bottom, pull your shoulders back and show the world a big broad chest.

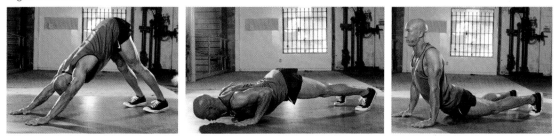

HIGH-KNEE SKIP

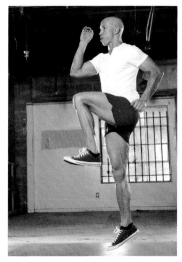

COOL-DOWN

ISOMETRIC PIGEON STRETCH
(8 x 10 seconds on each side)

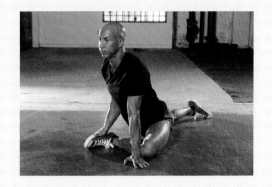

WARM-UP

Jumping Jacks (for sixty seconds)

Then do eight reps of each of these exercises, for two rounds total:

SIDE-LYING LEG LIFTS   ITB LEG LIFTS   BACKSTROKE

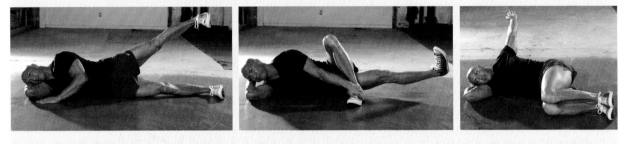

WORKOUT

50/10 WORK-TO-REST INTERVALS.

STRAIGHT LEG CRUNCH

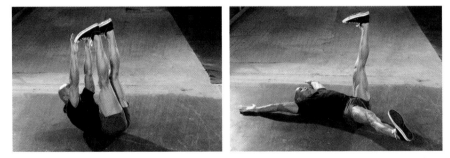

STRAIGHT LEG BRIDGE

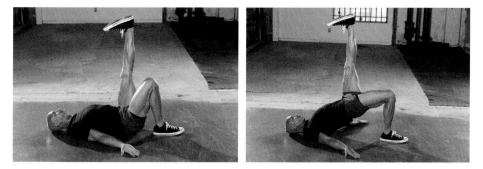

JUMP THRUST

TIP: Remember, to safely absorb the force of the landing, try to keep your feet parallel on landing, and immediately push your hips back as you land.

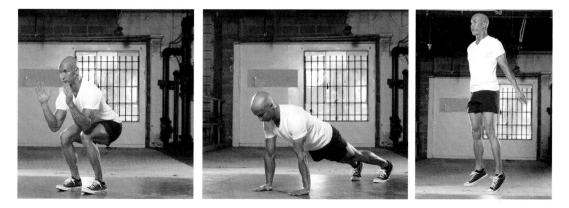

COOL-DOWN

HIP ROLLS *(eight slow reps)*

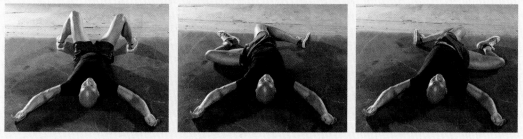

WARM-UP

Jumping Jacks (for sixty seconds)

Then do eight reps of each of these exercises, for two rounds total:

SIDE-LYING LEG LIFTS   ITB LEG LIFTS   BACKSTROKE

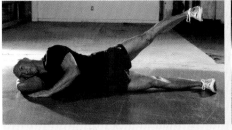 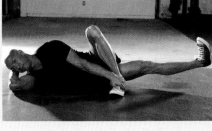 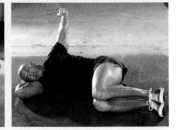

WORKOUT

50/10 WORK-TO-REST INTERVALS.

HIGH DROP

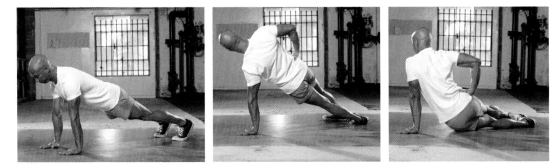

TRIPOD LET ME UPS

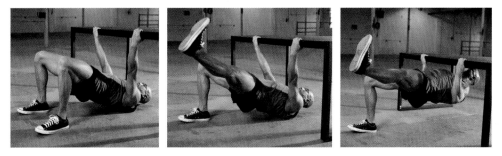

SIDE-TO-SIDE COSSACK

Hamstrings, glutes, quadriceps, hip rotators, hip flexors, spinal erectors, obliques, calves, shin muscles, deltoids, traps, abs, lats

From a tall double kneeling position, transition to single kneeling with your left leg forward. From there, get into a Cossack Squat with your left leg bent.

While keeping your hips low and chest up, shift to the right and get into a Cossack Squat with your right leg bent.

Take a brief moment in each end position to exhale fully, sink your hips, raise your chest, and fully straighten the extended leg. Continue switching side to side.

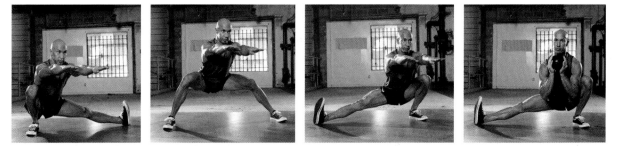

COOL-DOWN

SPIDERMAN A-FRAMES *(eight slow reps each side)*

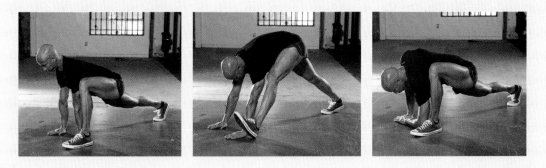

WARM-UP

March in Place (for sixty seconds)

Then do eight reps of each of these exercises, for two rounds total:

HIP CIRCLES   TWIST AND REACH   POINTERS

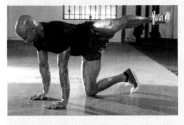
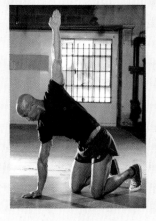
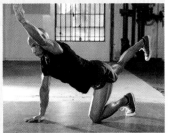

WORKOUT

50/10 WORK-TO-REST INTERVALS.

DIVE BOMBER

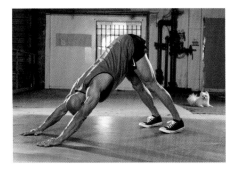
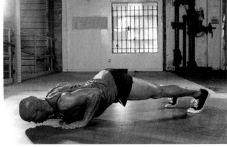
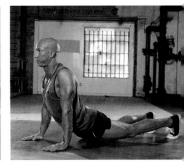

STRAIGHT LEG CRUNCH

TIP: Remember, as you lower your legs to the sides, keep the toes and knees pointing straight up. This is going to improve your control of the hip rotation, which has a major impact on how you move about in day-to-day life and actual sports. You don't need your knees and toes pointing outward when you're going straight ahead!

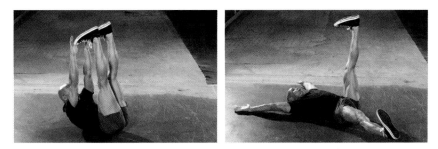

JUMP THRUST

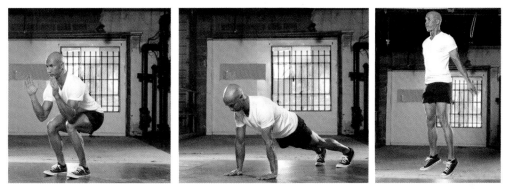

COOL-DOWN

SPIDERMAN ARM CIRCLES *(eight reps each side)*

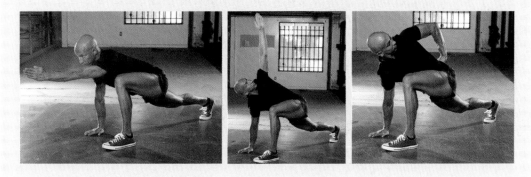

WARM-UP

March in Place (for sixty seconds)

Then do eight reps of each of these exercises, for two rounds total:

HIP CIRCLES   TWIST AND REACH   POINTERS

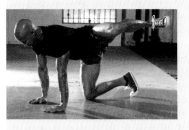
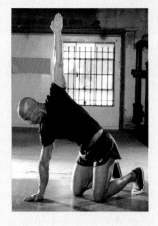
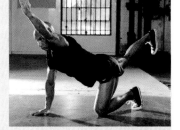

WORKOUT

50/10 WORK-TO-REST INTERVALS.

PARALLEL LEG BRIDGE

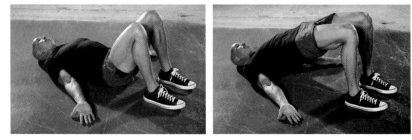

HIGH KICK

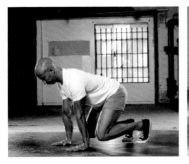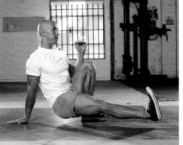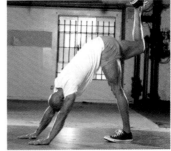

HIGH-KNEE SKIP

TIPS: Get your knees up as high as you can by aggressively stabbing your elbows straight back.

The backward motion of your arm swing helps to drive the opposite knee up higher.

Your lower hand should look like you're about to put your hand in your pocket.

The fingers of your upper hand should be at eyebrow height.

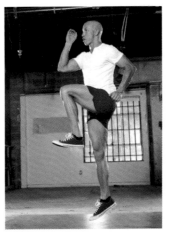

COOL-DOWN

BLOOMERS *(eight slow reps)*

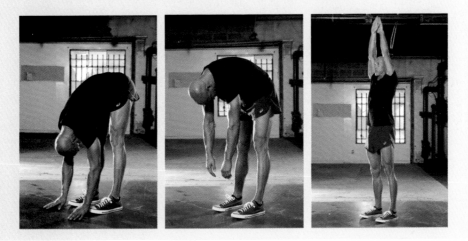

WARM-UP

March in Place (for sixty seconds)

Then do eight reps of each of these exercises, for two rounds total:

HIP CIRCLES   TWIST AND REACH   POINTERS

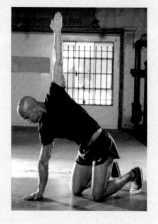

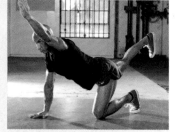

WORKOUT

50/10 WORK-TO-REST INTERVALS.

TRIPOD PRESS

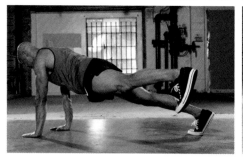

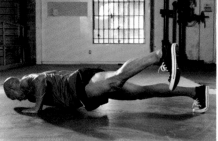

LET ME INS

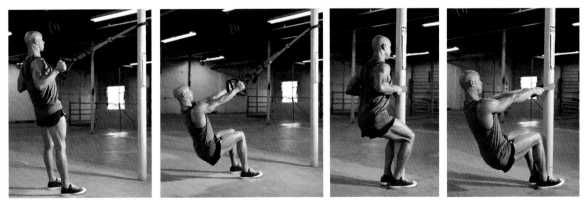

SIDE-TO-SIDE COSSACK (WEIGHTED OPTION)

Got a small dumbbell, kettlebell, or rock, or a backpack that you can throw some books in? Hold the weight to your chest as you do this exercise. The weight helps you to get into better positions, improving flexibility, strength, and endurance. Start light and progress gradually.

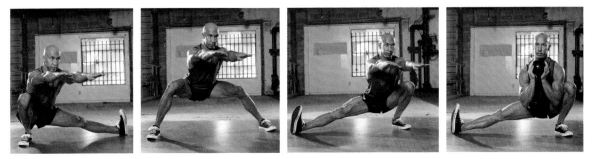

COOL-DOWN
STRADDLE REACH *(eight reps each side)*

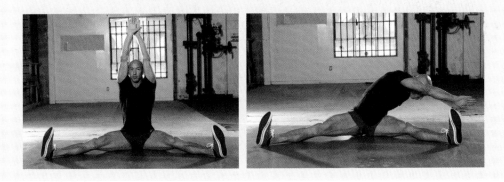

WARM-UP

March in Place (for sixty seconds)

Then do eight reps of each of these exercises, for two rounds total:

HIP CIRCLES   TWIST AND REACH   POINTERS

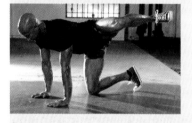 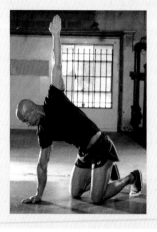 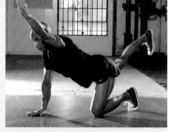

WORKOUT

50/10 WORK-TO-REST INTERVALS.

T-ARM REACH

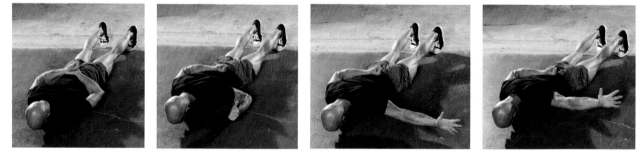

DOUBLE DROP

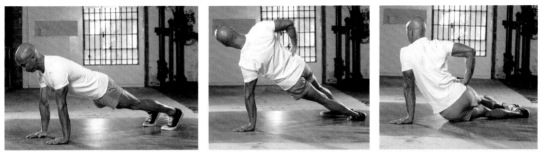

SQUAT TO ROMANIAN DEAD LIFT

TIP: Remember, stand up tall and straight after each rep, check the placement of your feet, and coordinate your breathing.

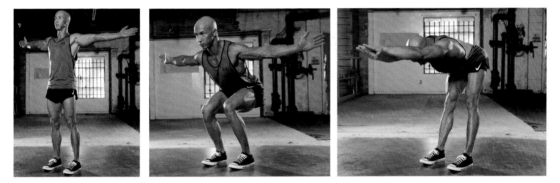

COOL-DOWN
ISOMETRIC PIGEON STRETCH
(8 x 10 seconds on each side)

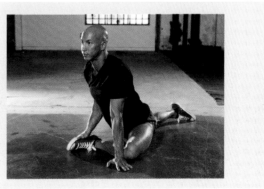

WARM-UP

March in Place (for sixty seconds)

Then do eight reps of each of these exercises, for two rounds total:

HIP CIRCLES   TWIST AND REACH   POINTERS

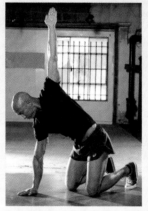
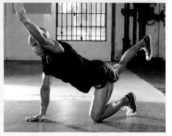

WORKOUT

50/10 WORK-TO-REST INTERVALS.

Y CUFF

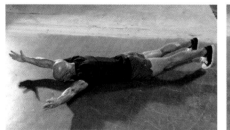
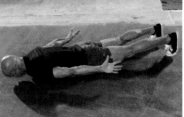
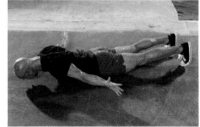

LOW DROP

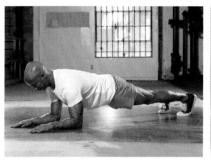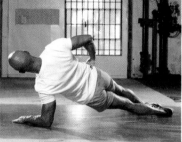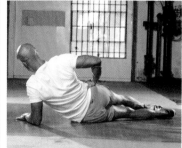

SQUAT THRUST

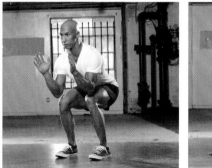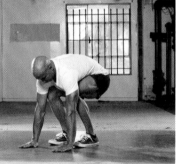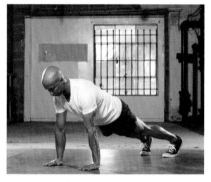

COOL-DOWN

HIP ROLLS *(eight slow reps)*

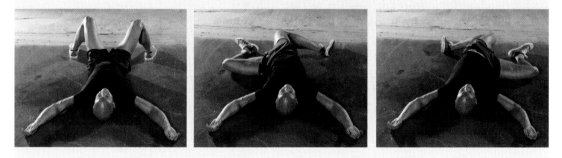

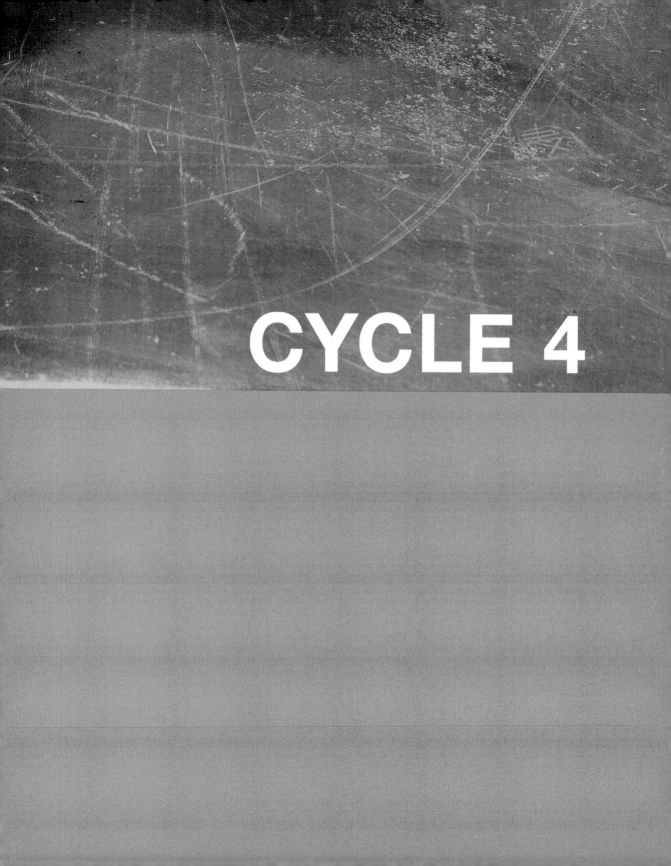

CYCLE 4

Never before has there been such a short-low-impact program that comprehensively and methodically covers all the muscle groups, joint functions, and athletic skills you require to get and stay strong, lean, healthy, mobile, and injury-free.

WARM-UP

Jumping Jacks (for sixty seconds)

Then do eight reps of each of these exercises, for two rounds total:

SIDE-LYING LEG LIFTS

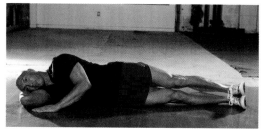

ITB LEG LIFTS

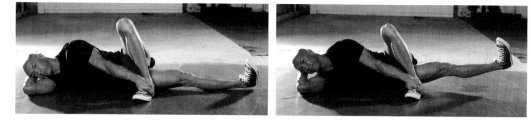

BACKSTROKE

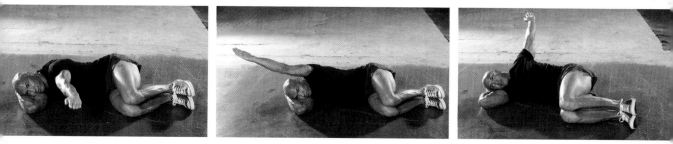

STARFISH DROP

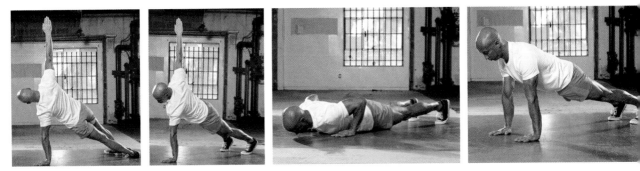

LET ME UPS

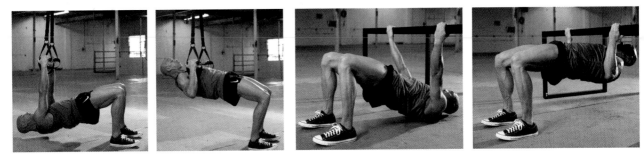

T-ARM SQUAT (WEIGHTED OPTION)

If you have a dumbbell, kettlebell, or any other weight, you can hold it to your chest as you do these squats. Everything is exactly the same except that you won't be holding your arms at the T position. Place your feet parallel and hip-to shoulder-width apart. Keep your knees pointed straight ahead. Push your hips straight back and lower your hips until your thighs are parallel to the floor. Keep your chest up in the bottom position.

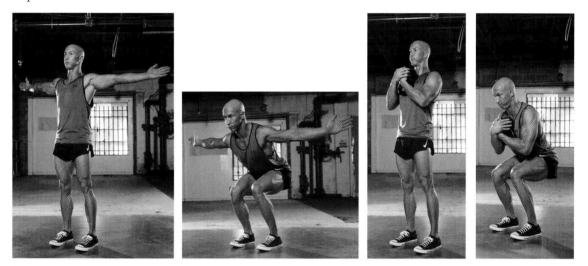

COOL-DOWN

SPIDERMAN A-FRAMES *(eight slow reps each side)*

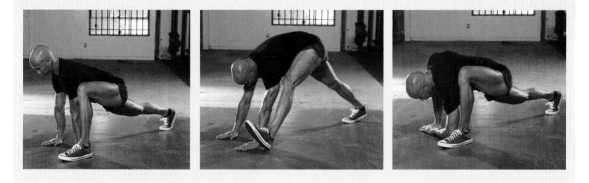

WARM-UP

March in Place (for sixty seconds)

Then do eight reps of each of these exercises, for two rounds total:

HIP CIRCLES   TWIST AND REACH   POINTERS

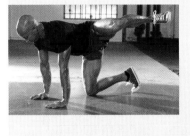
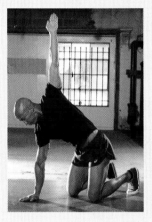
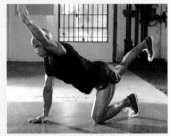

WORKOUT

40/20 WORK-TO-REST INTERVALS.

STRAIGHT LEG BRIDGE

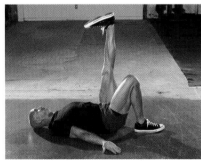
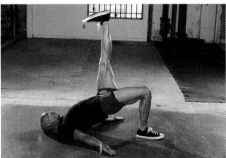

HIGH KICK

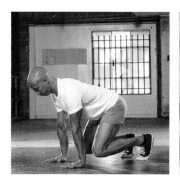 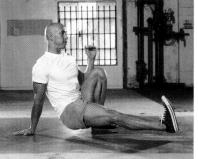 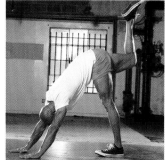

STORK STANCE

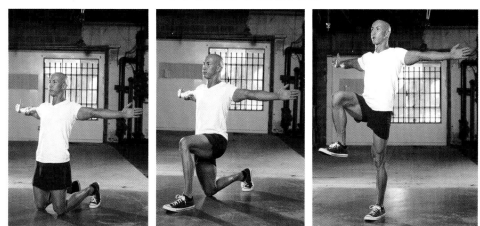

COOL-DOWN

SPIDERMAN ARM CIRCLES *(eight reps each side)*

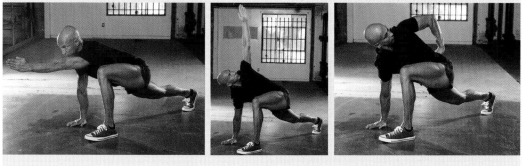

WARM-UP

Jumping Jacks (for sixty seconds)

Then do eight reps of each of these exercises, for two rounds total:

SIDE-LYING LEG LIFTS   ITB LEG LIFTS   BACKSTROKE

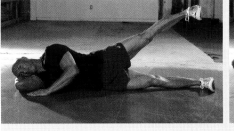 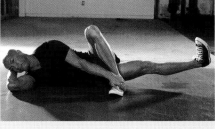 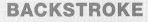 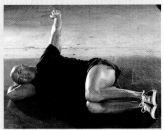

WORKOUT

60/00 WORK-TO-REST INTERVALS.

DOUBLE DROP

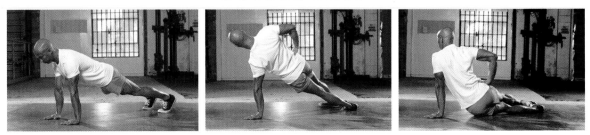

ALTERNATING GRIP PULL-UPS

Lats, rear deltoids, traps, biceps, forearms, spinal erectors, pectorals, glutes, quadriceps, hamstrings, shin muscles, abs

You need a Pull-Up bar, sturdy branch, or playfloor with monkey bars you can hang from. An inexpensive Pull-Up bar that anchors into a doorway is usually the easiest solution. If Pull-Ups aren't an option, do Let Me Ups or Let Me Ins.

With your left hand, grab the bar with your palm facing away from yourself. With your right hand, grab the bar with your palm facing toward you. Place your hands slightly wider than shoulder-width apart.

EXHALE: Pull yourself up as high as you can. Ideally, you want to clear your chin over the bar, but if you can't, that's totally fine.
INHALE: Lower yourself, and make yourself long and straight at the bottom. It's okay if you have to bend your knees to clear the floor.

Do two reps, then switch your grip. You are not expected to do this exercise nonstop. This is a good way to pace yourself. Doing just one rep at a time before letting go to change hand positions also works well to set a sustainable pace. Get a stretch at the end of each rep by coming to a full hang.

You can also do "negatives" where you cheat yourself up to the top, by jumping, stepping onto a chair, or getting someone to push you, and then control the way down, which should take three to five seconds.

If for some reason, you can't use an alternating grip, you can use an overhand or underhand grip. I like Alternating Grip Pull-Ups because you get the benefits of both hand positions in one exercise, and it's easier to hold on. Lastly, if none of these variations work for you, use Let Me Ups or Let Me Ins instead.

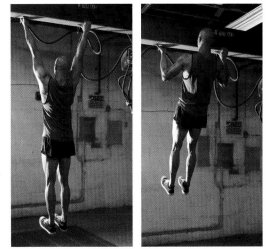

SIDE-TO-SIDE COSSACK (WEIGHTED OPTION)

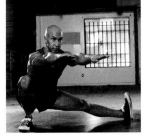 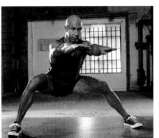 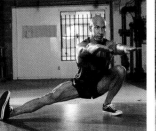 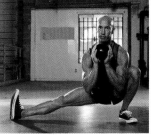

COOL-DOWN

BLOOMERS *(eight slow reps)*

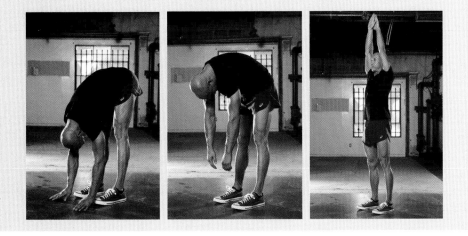

WARM-UP

March in Place (for sixty seconds)

Then do eight reps of each of these exercises, for two rounds total:

HIP CIRCLES   TWIST AND REACH   POINTERS

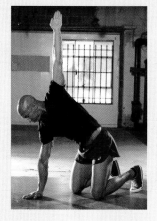
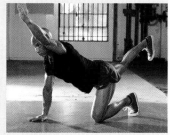

WORKOUT

40/20 WORK-TO-REST INTERVALS.

BENT LEG BRIDGE

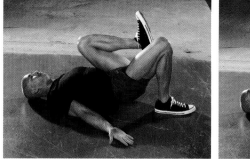
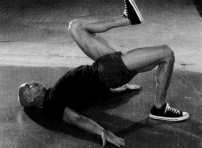

ARM HAULERS

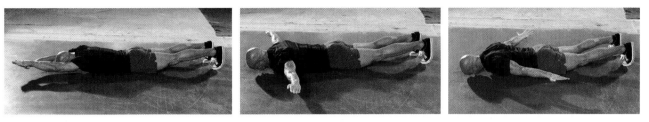

HIGH-KNEE MARCH

TIPS: Remember, fully extend through the supporting leg, and get your knees up high by stabbing your elbows straight back behind yourself. Also, keep your midsection tight to prevent your back from arching.

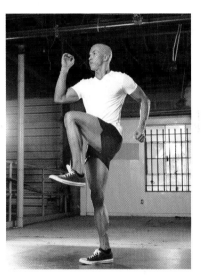

COOL-DOWN

STRADDLE REACH *(eight reps each side)*

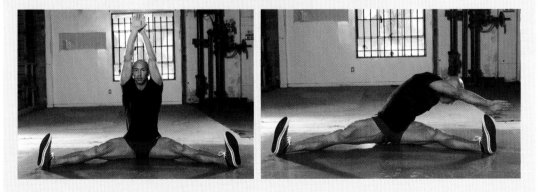

WARM-UP

Jumping Jacks (for sixty seconds)

Then do eight reps of each of these exercises, for two rounds total:.

SIDE-LYING LEG LIFTS   ITB LEG LIFTS   BACKSTROKE

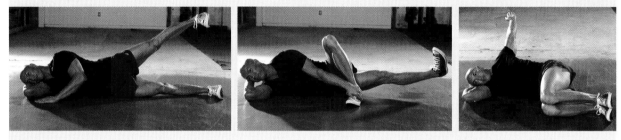

WORKOUT

60/00 WORK-TO-REST INTERVALS.

DIVE BOMBER

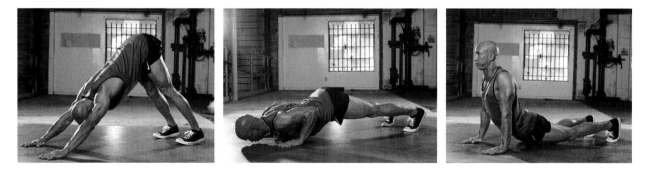

LET ME INS

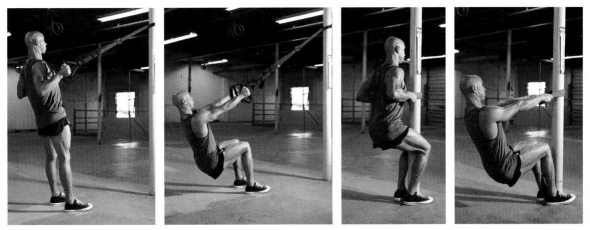

T-ARM SQUAT (WEIGHTED OPTION)

You can do this exercise while holding a weight to your chest.

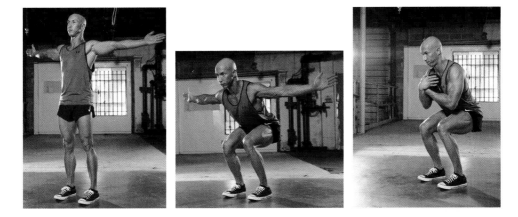

COOL-DOWN

ISOMETRIC
PIGEON STRETCH

(8 x 10 seconds on each side)

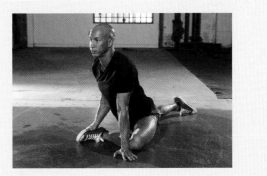

WARM-UP

March in Place (for sixty seconds)

Then do eight reps of each of these exercises, for two rounds total:

HIP CIRCLES   TWIST AND REACH   POINTERS

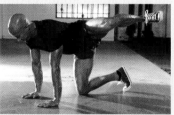
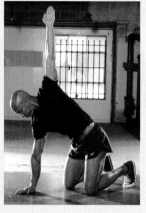
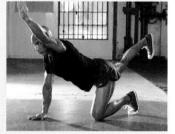

WORKOUT

40/20 WORK-TO-REST INTERVALS.

STRAIGHT LEG CRUNCH

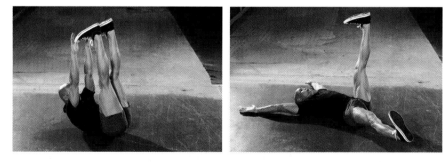

STARFISH TWIST

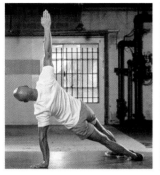 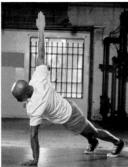 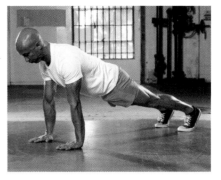

HIGH-KNEE RUN

TIP: Fully extend through the leg that's in contact with the floor, while aggressively stabbing the opposite elbow straight back to get the knee of the opposite leg as high as you can. Keep your midsection tight, and lean forward slightly. Focus more on high knees and less on speed.

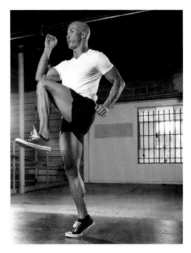

COOL-DOWN

HIP ROLLS *(eight slow reps)*

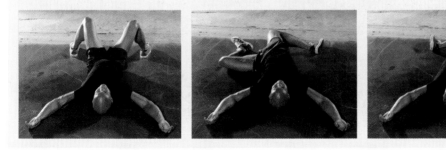

WARM-UP

Jumping Jacks (for sixty seconds)

Then do eight reps of each of these exercises, for two rounds total:

SIDE-LYING LEG LIFTS   ITB LEG LIFTS   BACKSTROKE

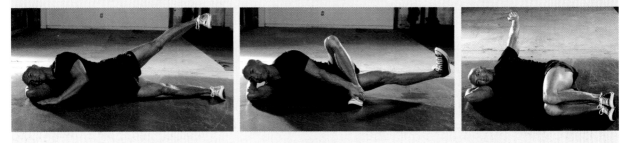

WORKOUT

40/20 WORK-TO-REST INTERVALS.

DIVE BOMBER

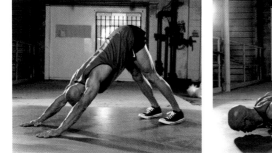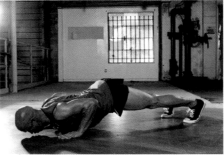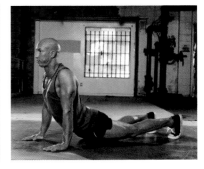

ALTERNATING GRIP PULL-UPS

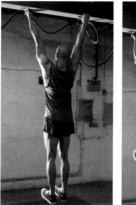
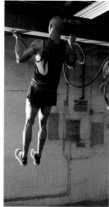

STREAMLINE BULGARIAN SPLIT SQUAT

Hamstrings, glutes, quadriceps, hip rotators, hip flexors, spinal erectors, deltoids, traps, abs, obliques, calves, shin muscles, lats, triceps, neck

Find a sturdy chair or other surface that's knee height or slightly lower. Stand in front of the surface as if you're about to sit on it. Take a normal-size step forward with the left foot and place your right foot on the chair. Bring your arms overhead to the streamline positions and tighten your abdominals as if someone might punch you in the gut.

INHALE: Sink your hips back and down as far as you can.
EXHALE: Reset to a tall standing position on one leg.

Continue on the same leg until you hit the thirty-second mark. Then quickly switch legs and complete the remaining thirty-second interval.

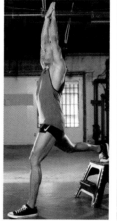
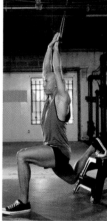

COOL-DOWN

SPIDERMAN A-FRAMES *(eight slow reps each side)*

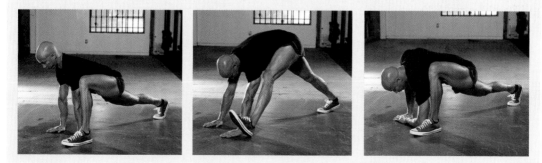

WARM-UP

March in Place (for sixty seconds)

Then do eight reps of each of these exercises, for two rounds total:

HIP CIRCLES   TWIST AND REACH   POINTERS

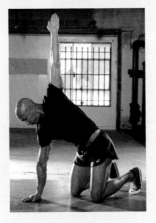

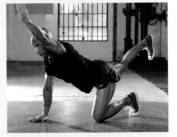

WORKOUT

60/00 WORK-TO-REST INTERVALS.

BENT LEG BRIDGE

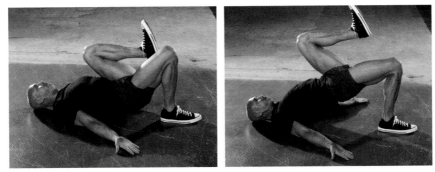

LOW DROP

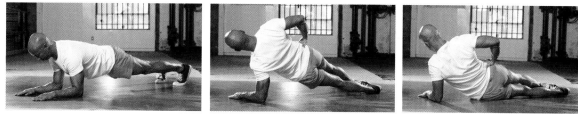

HIGH-KNEE RUN

TIP: As the raised knee comes down, the other knee should already be coming up.

The difference between the High-Knee March and High-Knee Run is that for marching, one foot is always in contact with the floor. For running, the planted foot comes up as the raised foot comes down. And that's actually also one of the main differences between regular walking and running. Running has a "flight phase."

You can skip using both of these techniques, but the latter is more athletic.

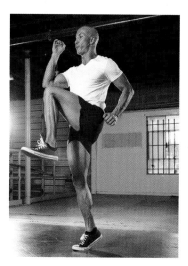

COOL-DOWN

SPIDERMAN ARM CIRCLES *(eight reps each side)*

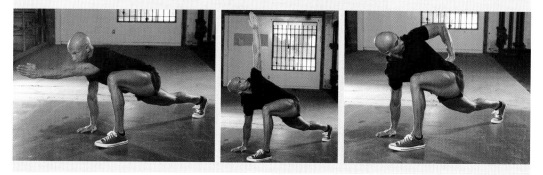

WARM-UP

Jumping Jacks (for sixty seconds)

Then do eight reps of each of these exercises, for two rounds total:

SIDE-LYING LEG LIFTS   ITB LEG LIFTS   BACKSTROKE

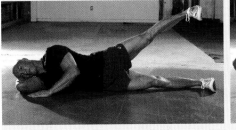 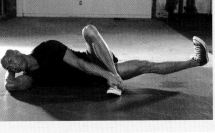 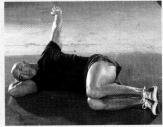

WORKOUT

60/00 WORK-TO-REST INTERVALS.

DOUBLE FUN GLIDE

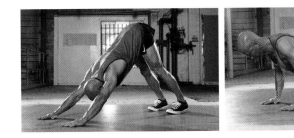 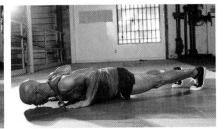

TRIPOD LET ME UPS

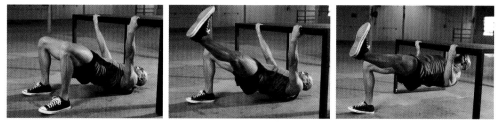

STREAMLINE ROMANIAN DEAD LIFT
(WEIGHTED OPTION)

If you have a dumbbell, kettlebell, or any other compact weighted object, you can hold it high up against your chest as shown in the images. If you use a weight, your arms won't be at the streamline position, but everything else is the same.

Your feet are hip- to shoulder-width apart and parallel. Push your hips straight back and hip hinge forward with a straight back and straight legs.

Once you feel the stretch, reverse the movement. The flexibility of your hamstrings determines how far you can go while keeping your back straight. If it isn't very far, don't worry, it'll get better, especially if you can learn to keep your legs and back straight while doing this movement.

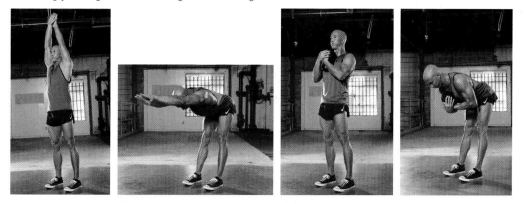

COOL-DOWN
BLOOMERS *(eight slow reps)*

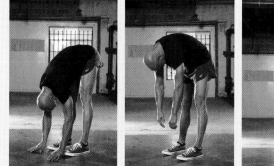

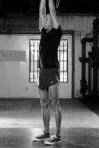

WARM-UP

March in Place (for sixty seconds)

Then do eight reps of each of these exercises, for two rounds total:

HIP CIRCLES   TWIST AND REACH   POINTERS

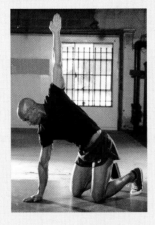
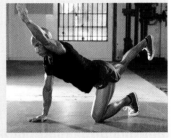

WORKOUT

40/20 WORK-TO-REST INTERVALS.

T-ARM REACH

TIP: Keep your glutes flexed, belly button drawn in toward your spine, and your chin slightly tucked.

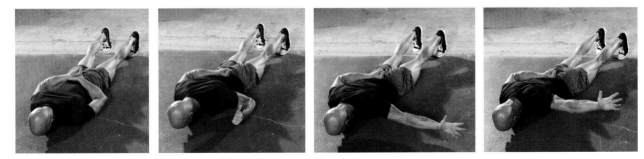

STRAIGHT LEG BRIDGE

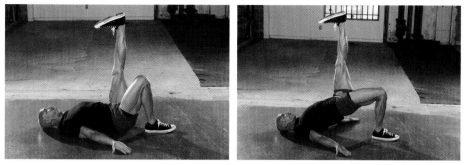

PARALLEL LEG CRUNCH

TIPS: At the bottom of each rep, reach as far as you can to the Y position past your head while exhaling and keeping your lower back in contact with the floor.

Challenging your shoulder mobility in this way also challenges your posture (and so builds the most strength), since we have the tendency to arch our backs when we reach past our heads.

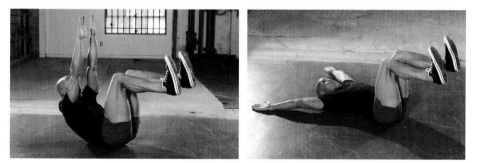

COOL-DOWN

STRADDLE REACH *(eight reps each side)*

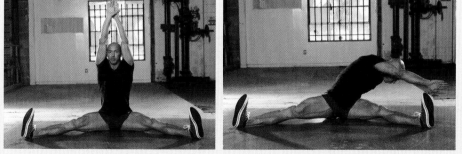

WARM-UP

Jumping Jacks (for sixty seconds)

Then do eight reps of each of these exercises, for two rounds total:

SIDE-LYING LEG LIFTS   ITB LEG LIFTS   BACKSTROKE

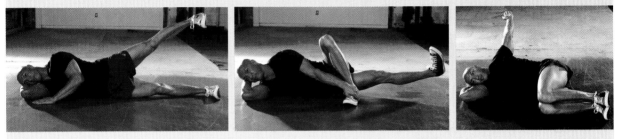

WORKOUT

60/00 WORK-TO-REST INTERVALS.

TRIPOD PRESS

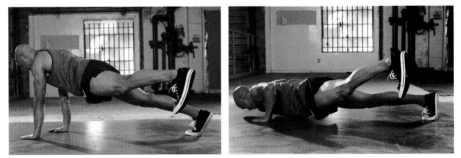

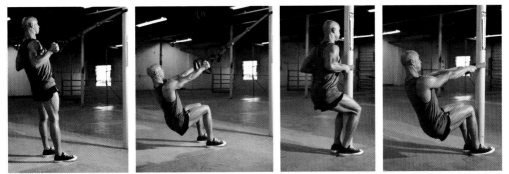

ROMANIAN DEAD LIFT TO SQUAT (WEIGHTED OPTION)

This is another wonderful exercise that can be done while holding a weight high up on your chest.

Everything except the arm positions remains the same. Keep your feet hip- to shoulder-width apart and parallel. Make your legs straight for the dead lift portion, and lift your chest up in the bottom of the Squat.

Keep your back straight throughout this exercise!

Start light. Progress gradually.

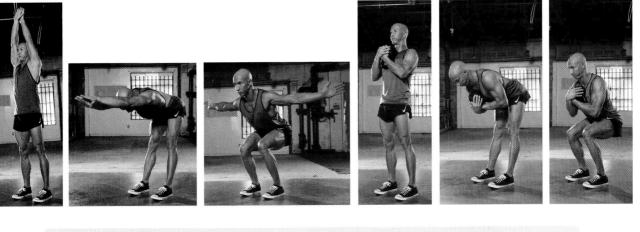

COOL-DOWN

ISOMETRIC PIGEON STRETCH

(8 x 10 seconds on each side)

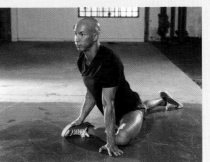

WARM-UP

March in Place (for sixty seconds)

Then do eight reps of each of these exercises, for two rounds total:

HIP CIRCLES   TWIST AND REACH   POINTERS

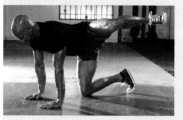 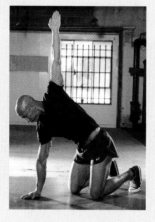 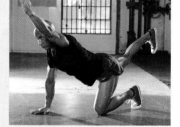

WORKOUT

45/15 WORK-TO-REST INTERVALS.

BENT LEG BRIDGE

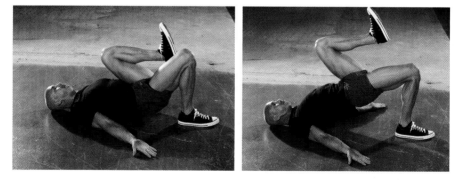

HIGH DROP

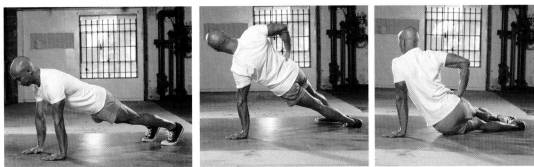

SIDE SQUAT

TIP: Remember, in each Side Squat position, get your feet parallel to each other with the bent knee pointing in the same direction as your toes, and keep your chest up.

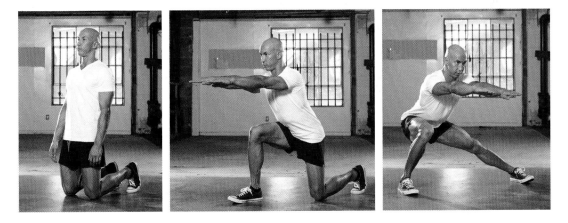

COOL-DOWN

HIP ROLLS *(eight slow reps)*

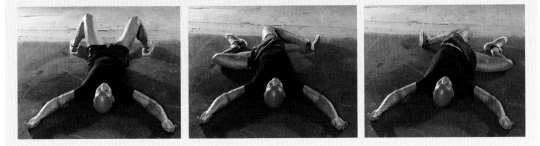

WARM-UP

Jumping Jacks (for sixty seconds)

Then do eight reps of each of these exercises, for two rounds total:

SIDE-LYING LEG LIFTS   ITB LEG LIFTS   BACKSTROKE

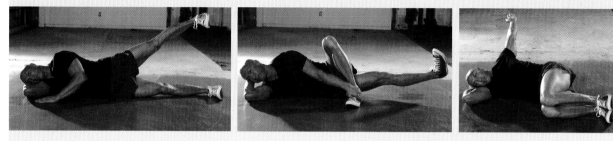

WORKOUT

60/00 WORK-TO-REST INTERVALS.

SIDE KICK

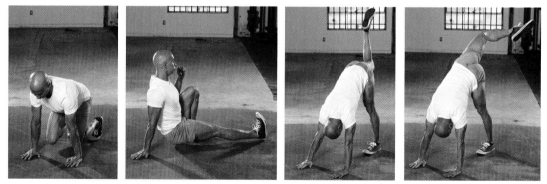

ALTERNATING GRIP PULL-UPS

TIPS: Make yourself long in the bottom position after each rep and get a good stretch. Take your time. It's okay to take short rests after every rep or every other rep.

Let Me Ups or Let Me Ins are acceptable replacements if you can't do Pull-Ups.

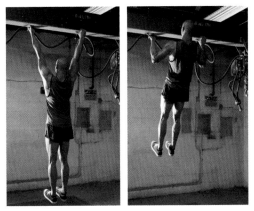

STREAMLINE BULGARIAN SPLIT SQUAT (WEIGHTED OPTION)

Holding a light weight to your chest as shown will help you get in a deeper split Squat, which will strengthen and stretch your hip flexors, which is vital, especially if you sit a lot.

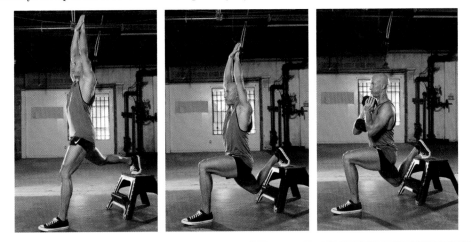

COOL-DOWN

SPIDERMAN A-FRAMES *(eight slow reps each side)*

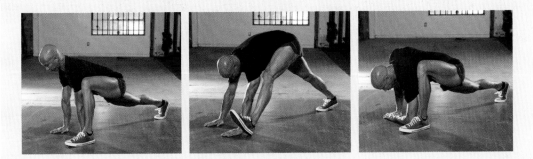

WARM-UP

March in Place (for sixty seconds)

Then do eight reps of each of these exercises, for two rounds total:

HIP CIRCLES   TWIST AND REACH   POINTERS

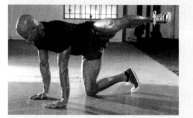 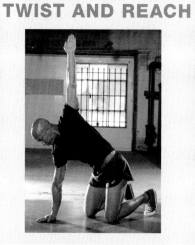 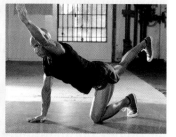

WORKOUT

45/15 WORK-TO-REST INTERVALS.

LOW DROP

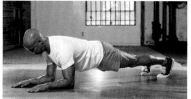 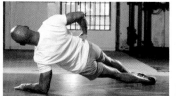 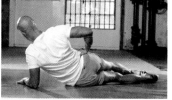

HIGH-KNEE MARCH

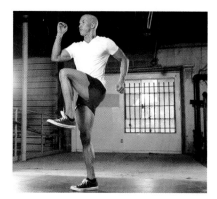

STORK STANCE

TIPS: Remember, stand up tall and straight every rep by fully extending the bottom leg, lifting your chest slightly, and tightening your abs. Get your knee up, and dorsiflex the raised ankle.

Think of this exercise as a slow version of the High-Knee Drills to get you into better positions for those exercises, which have a very practical carry-over to common real-life activities like walking, jogging, and sprinting.

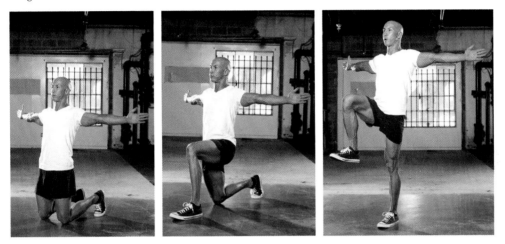

COOL-DOWN

SPIDERMAN ARM CIRCLES *(eight reps each side)*

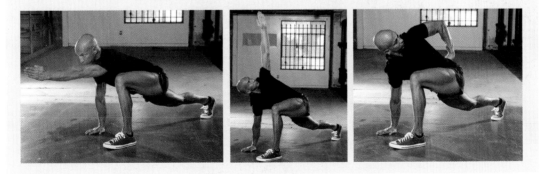

WARM-UP

Jumping Jacks (for sixty seconds)

Then do eight reps of each of these exercises, for two rounds total:

SIDE-LYING LEG LIFTS   ITB LEG LIFTS   BACKSTROKE

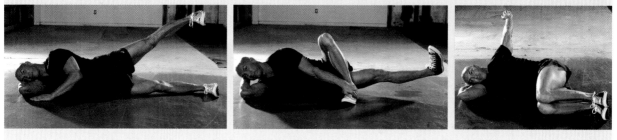

WORKOUT

60/00 WORK-TO-REST INTERVALS.

DOUBLE FUN GLIDE

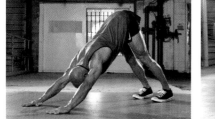
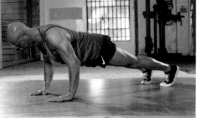
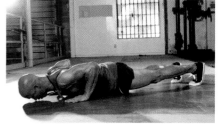

LET ME UPS

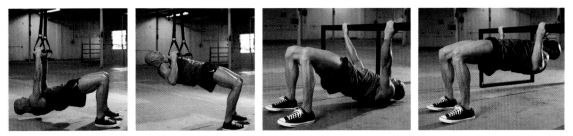

BOTTOM SQUAT (WEIGHTED OPTION)

You can try doing this exercise while holding a weight to your chest. Start light.

Keep your hips low and chest up as you transition in and out of the Bottom Squat. Your feet should be parallel to each other and about hip-width apart.

In the Bottom Squat, keep your knees pointing straight ahead.

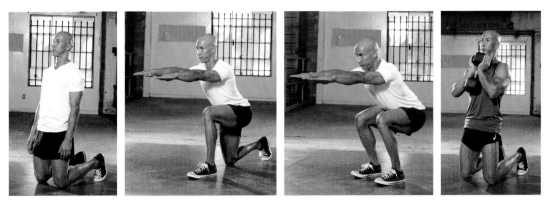

COOL-DOWN

BLOOMERS *(eight slow reps)*

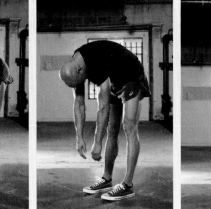
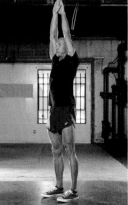

WARM-UP

March in Place (for sixty seconds)

Then do eight reps of each of these exercises, for two rounds total:

HIP CIRCLES   TWIST AND REACH   POINTERS

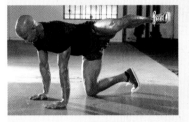
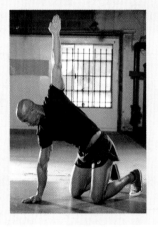
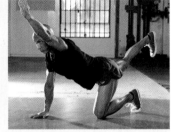

WORKOUT

45/15 WORK-TO-REST INTERVALS.

T-ARM REACH

TIP: Keep your chest on the floor as you do this exercise.

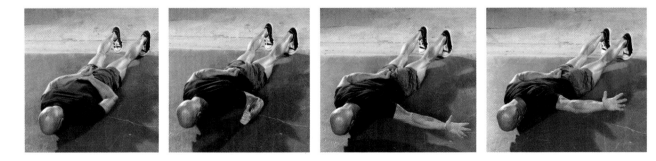

KICKOUT

TIP: Lift your chest and exhale in the Kickout positions.

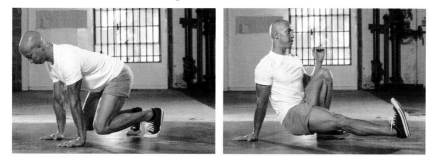

HIGH-KNEE SKIP

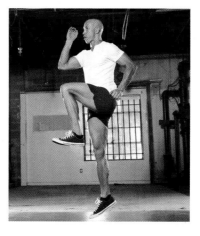

COOL-DOWN

STRADDLE REACH *(eight reps each side)*

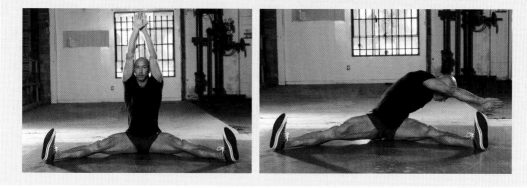

WARM-UP

Jumping Jacks (for sixty seconds)

Then do eight reps of each of these exercises, for two rounds total:

SIDE-LYING LEG LIFTS   ITB LEG LIFTS   BACKSTROKE

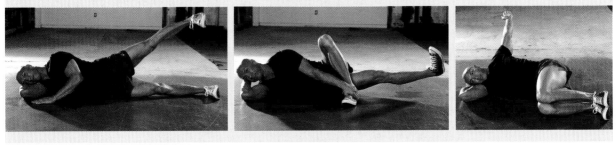

WORKOUT

60/00 WORK-TO-REST INTERVALS.

TRIPOD PRESS

TIP: Dorsiflex the elevated ankle, and keep your feet parallel with your elevated knee and toes pointing down.

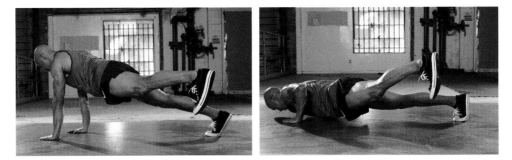

TRIPOD LET ME UPS

TIP: Similar to the Tripod Press, control hip rotation by keeping the knee and toes of the raised leg pointing up.

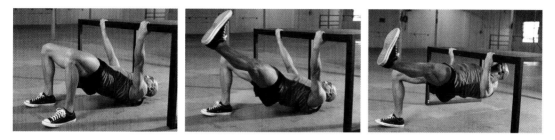

SIDE-TO-SIDE COSSACK (WEIGHTED OPTION)

TIP: Point the toes and knee of the extended leg straight up.

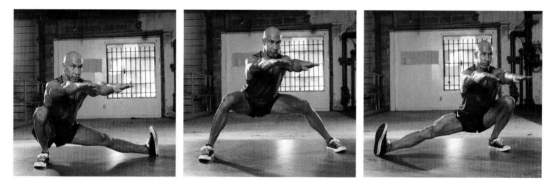

COOL-DOWN
ISOMETRIC PIGEON STRETCH
(8 x 10 seconds on each side)

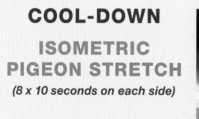
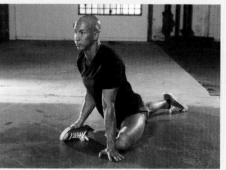

WARM-UP

March in Place (for sixty seconds)

Then do eight reps of each of these exercises, for two rounds total:

HIP CIRCLES   TWIST AND REACH   POINTERS

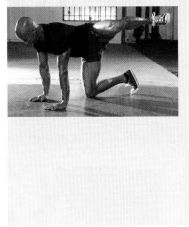
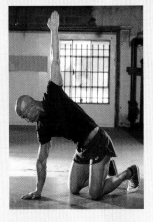
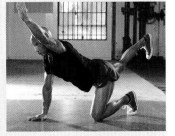

WORKOUT

45/15 WORK-TO-REST INTERVALS.

PARALLEL LEG CRUNCH

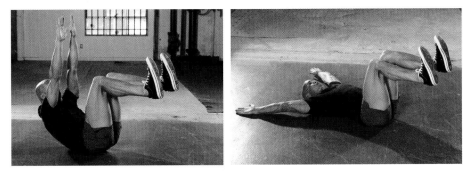

HIGH-KNEE MARCH

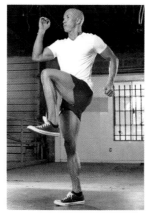

STREAMLINE ROMANIAN DEAD LIFT

TIP: In the bottom position, when you're feeling a stretch in your hamstrings, take a brief moment to push your hips back and reach forward with your arms. Challenge yourself to get as long as possible. Then stand up tall and straight.

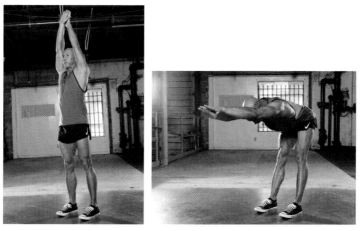

COOL-DOWN

HIP ROLLS *(eight slow reps)*

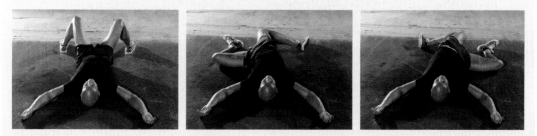

WARM-UP

Jumping Jacks (for sixty seconds)

Then do eight reps of each of these exercises, for two rounds total:

| SIDE-LYING LEG LIFTS | ITB LEG LIFTS | BACKSTROKE |

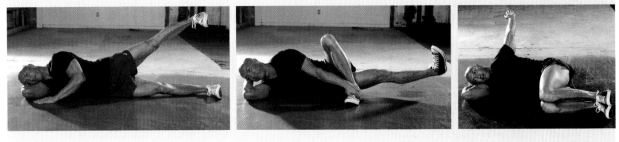

WORKOUT

60/00 WORK-TO-REST INTERVALS.

DOUBLE FUN GLIDE

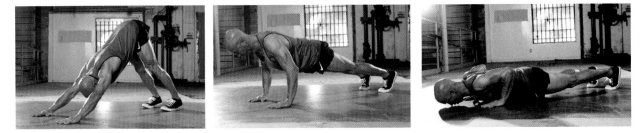

ALTERNATING GRIP PULL-UPS

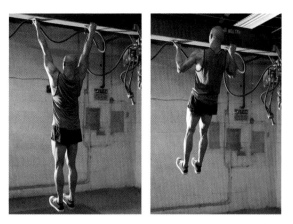

SQUAT TO ROMANIAN DEAD LIFT (WEIGHTED OPTION)

If you have a small weight, hold it high up against your chest while doing this exercise, as shown.

Your feet should be hip-to shoulder-width apart and parallel to each other. Everything is the same using a weight except the arm positions. Be sure to stand up tall and straight after every rep, and take the time to get into the best possible positions for the Squat and Romanian Dead Lift.

If you don't have a weight, use the T-Arm Squat and Streamline Romanian Deadlift arm positions.

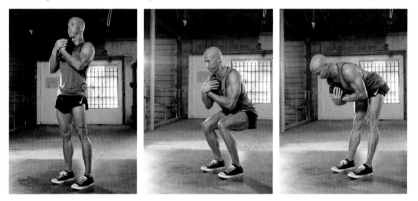

COOL-DOWN

SPIDERMAN A-FRAMES *(eight slow reps each side)*

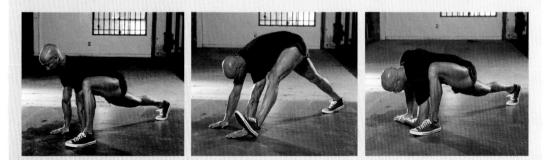

WARM-UP

March in Place (for sixty seconds)

Then do eight reps of each of these exercises, for two rounds total:

HIP CIRCLES   TWIST AND REACH   POINTERS

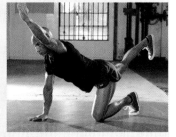
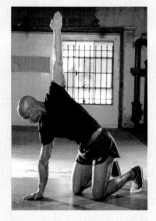
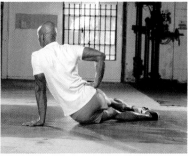

WORKOUT

45/15 WORK-TO-REST INTERVALS.

DOUBLE DROP

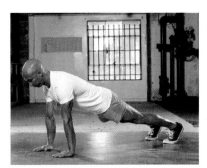
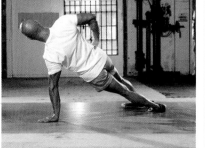
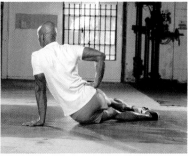

HIGH-KNEE RUN

TIP: I want you to push hard on these runs. Remember, the world record 400-meter dash is 43.03 seconds! Think about beating that!

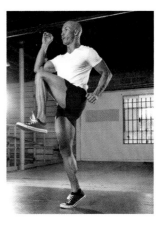

JUMP THRUST

TIP: Stay relaxed and focus on your form.

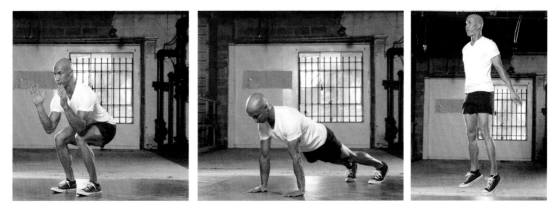

COOL-DOWN

SPIDERMAN ARM CIRCLES *(eight reps each side)*

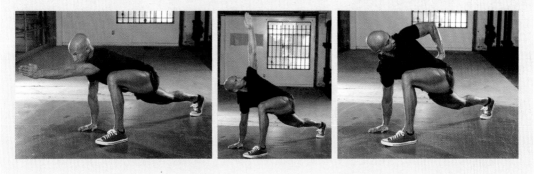

WARM-UP

Jumping Jacks (for sixty seconds)

Then do eight reps of each of these exercises, for two rounds total:

SIDE-LYING LEG LIFTS   ITB LEG LIFTS   BACKSTROKE

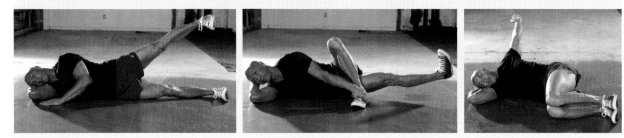

WORKOUT

60/00 WORK-TO-REST INTERVALS.

STARFISH BOUNCE

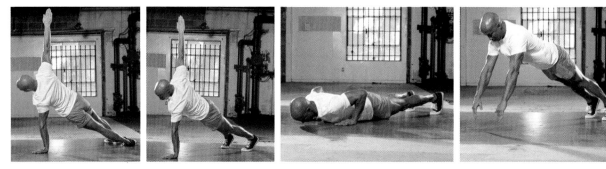

TRIPOD LET ME UPS

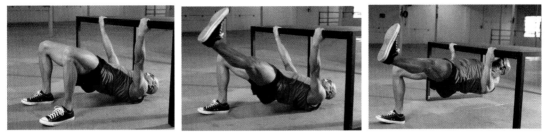

SIDE SQUAT (WEIGHTED OPTION)

If you have a light weight, hold it to your chest while doing this exercise.

Keep your hips low and chest up in the Side Squat position. Your feet should be parallel with the bent knee pointing in the same direction as your feet.

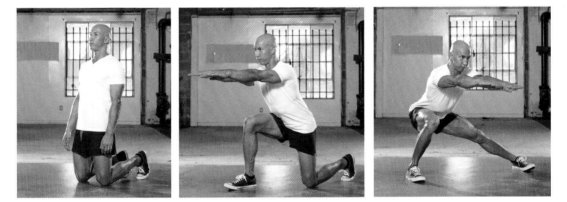

COOL-DOWN

BLOOMERS *(eight slow reps)*

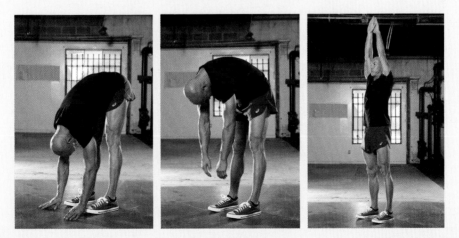

WARM-UP

March in Place (for sixty seconds)

Then do eight reps of each of these exercises, for two rounds total:

HIP CIRCLES   TWIST AND REACH   POINTERS

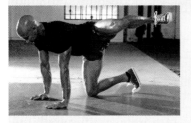
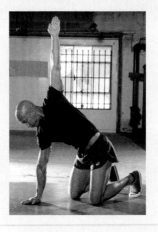
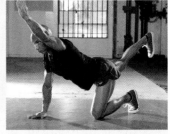

WORKOUT

50/10 WORK-TO-REST INTERVALS.

BENT LEG CRUNCH

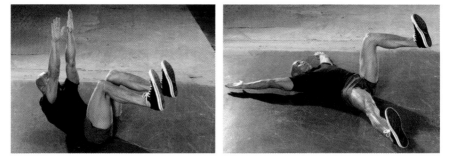

SIDE KICK

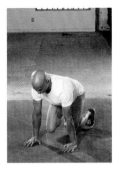 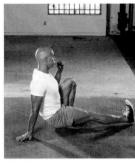 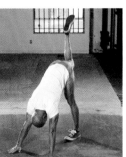 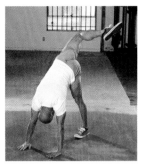

ROMANIAN DEAD LIFT TO SQUAT

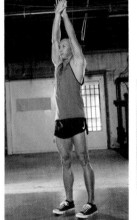

TIP: Remember, make your arms perfectly straight as you transition between the Streamline Romanian Deadlift and T-Arm Squat. Fully extend through your fingertips as if lightning bolts are coming out of them.

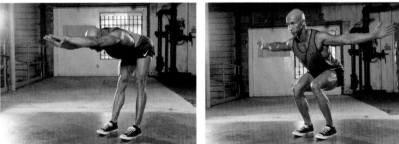

COOL-DOWN

STRADDLE REACH *(eight reps each side)*

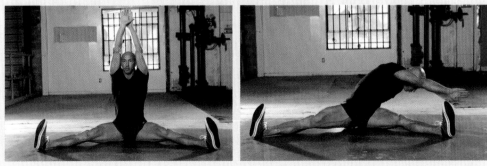

WARM-UP

Jumping Jacks (for sixty seconds)

Then do eight reps of each of these exercises, for two rounds total:

SIDE-LYING LEG LIFTS   ITB LEG LIFTS   BACKSTROKE

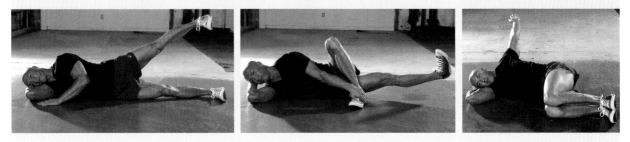

WORKOUT

60/00 WORK-TO-REST INTERVALS.

DIVE BOMBER

TIP: Remember, at the top of each rep, fully straighten your legs, let your heels sink to the floor, and push your chest down toward your feet to get a good stretch.

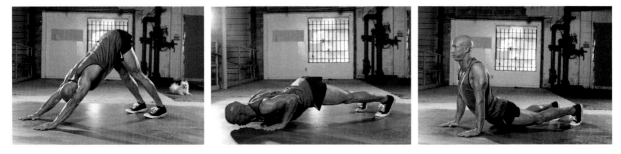

ALTERNATING GRIP PULL-UPS

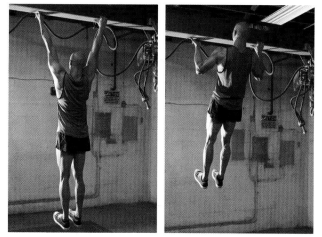

STREAMLINE BULGARIAN SPLIT SQUAT
(WEIGHTED OPTION)

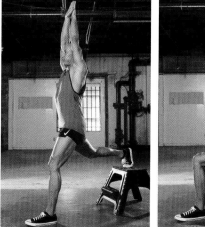
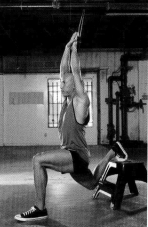

COOL-DOWN

ISOMETRIC
PIGEON STRETCH

(8 x 10 seconds on each side)

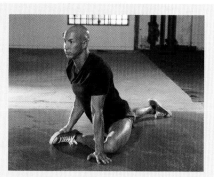

WARM-UP

March in Place (for sixty seconds)

Then do eight reps of each of these exercises, for two rounds total:

HIP CIRCLES   TWIST AND REACH   POINTERS

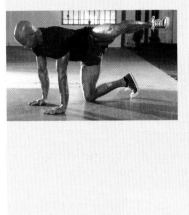 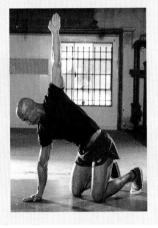 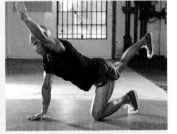

WORKOUT

50/10 WORK-TO-REST INTERVALS.

STRAIGHT LEG CRUNCH

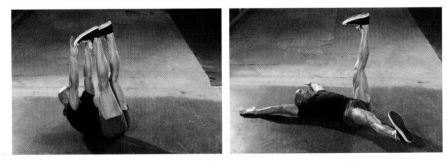

HIGH-KNEE SKIP

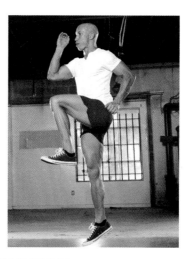

DROP THRUST

TIPS: Focus on making yourself perfectly straight as you kick your legs back and drop into the bottom of the Push-Up. Also, make sure you're transitioning in and out of a perfect Squat. You'll build more strength that way, as well as habits that will keep you injury-free throughout the rest of the day.

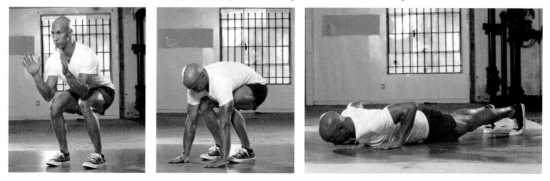

COOL-DOWN

HIP ROLLS *(eight slow reps)*

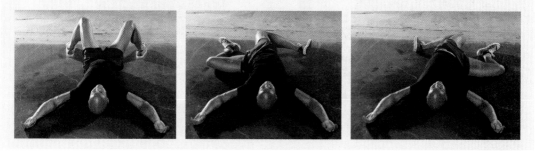

WARM-UP

Jumping Jacks (for sixty seconds)

Then do eight reps of each of these exercises, for two rounds total:

SIDE-LYING LEG LIFTS   ITB LEG LIFTS   BACKSTROKE

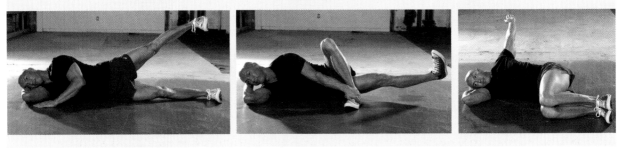

WORKOUT

60/00 WORK-TO-REST INTERVALS.

TRIPOD PRESS

TIPS: Lower yourself fully so that you're lying on the floor before pushing yourself back up.

Make yourself straight as an arrow at the top of each rep and on the way down. Try to hold that position on the way up, but if you can't, it's okay to worm yourself up and then focus on keeping your form perfect for the negative portion of the movement as you return to the floor.

The position of your body is far more important than the number of reps you do!

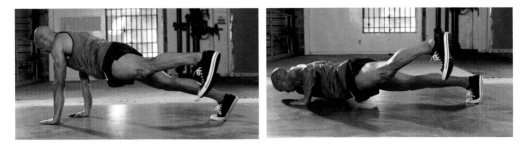

LET ME INS

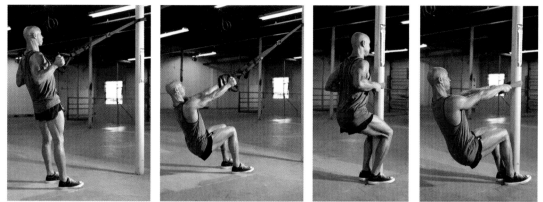

SIDE-TO-SIDE COSSACK (WEIGHTED OPTION)

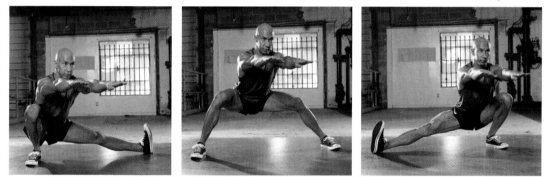

COOL-DOWN

SPIDERMAN A-FRAMES *(eight slow reps each side)*

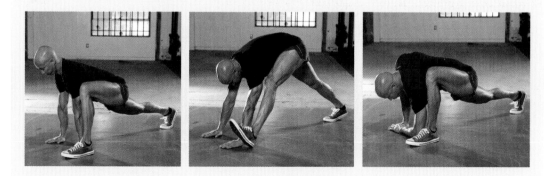

WARM-UP

March in Place (for sixty seconds)

Then do eight reps of each of these exercises, for two rounds total:

HIP CIRCLES   TWIST AND REACH   POINTERS

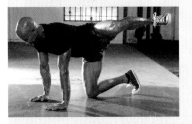 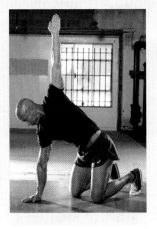 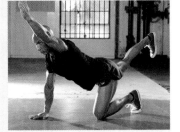

WORKOUT

50/10 WORK-TO-REST INTERVALS.

Y CUFF

TIP: Remember, reach as far as possible to the Y position while exhaling, tensing your glutes, and drawing your navel in toward your spine.

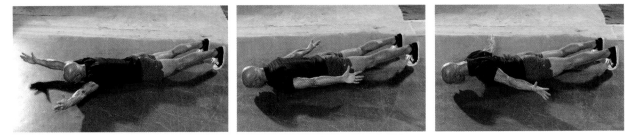

BENT LEG CRUNCH

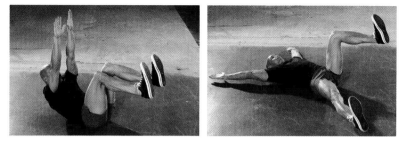

T-ARM SQUAT

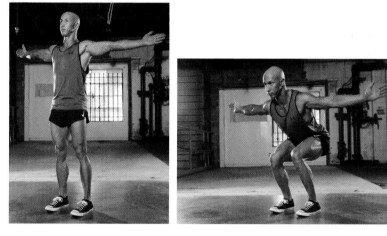

COOL-DOWN

SPIDERMAN ARM CIRCLES *(eight reps each side)*

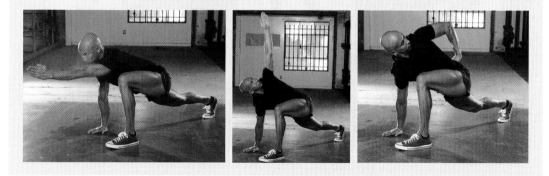

WARM-UP

Jumping Jacks (for sixty seconds)

Then do eight reps of each of these exercises, for two rounds total:

SIDE-LYING LEG LIFTS   ITB LEG LIFTS   BACKSTROKE

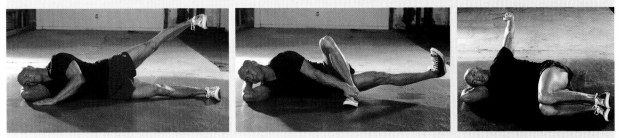

WORKOUT

60/00 WORK-TO-REST INTERVALS.

TRIPOD PRESS

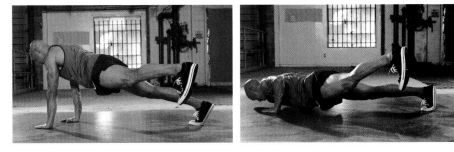

ALTERNATING GRIP PULL-UPS

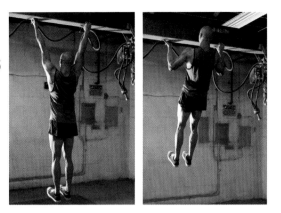

STORK STANCE (WEIGHTED OPTION)

This is another great exercise where holding a weight to your chest does wonders. Keep your chest up and midsection tight. Make yourself tall in the kneeling and standing positions. Transition between double kneeling, single kneeling, and Stork Stance with big steps!

Weight shifting with an extra load is possibly the most effective way to improve overall strength and stability, because we use side-to-side weight shifting for just about everything—like walking, running, striking, throwing, and so on. And Stork Stance develops this by eliminating unnecessary movement.

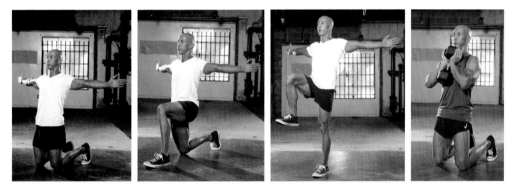

COOL-DOWN
BLOOMERS *(eight slow reps)*

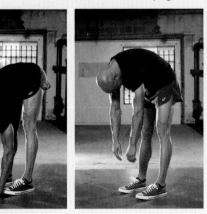
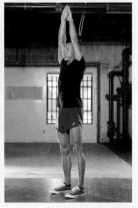

WARM-UP

March in Place (for sixty seconds)

Then do eight reps of each of these exercises, for two rounds total:

HIP CIRCLES   TWIST AND REACH   POINTERS

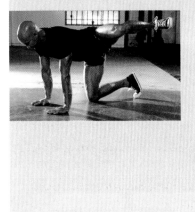
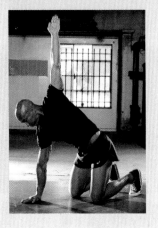
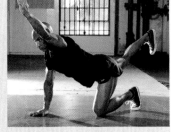

WORKOUT

50/10 WORK-TO-REST INTERVALS.

T-ARM REACH

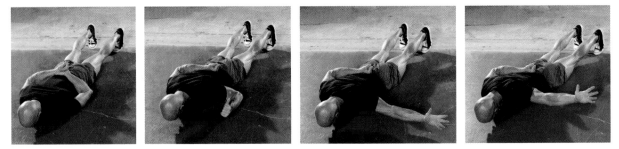

HIGH-KNEE SKIP

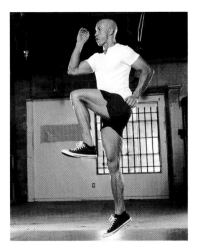

ROMANIAN DEAD LIFT TO SQUAT

TIPS: Coordinate your breathing! Inhale as you bend forward; exhale forcefully as you sink into the Squat.

Inhale as you transition back to the bottom of the Romanian Dead Lift, and exhale fully as you stand up tall and straight.

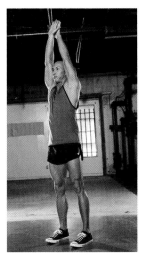
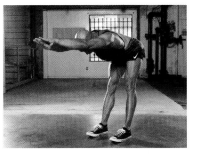
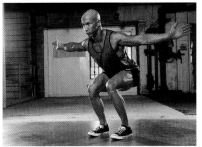

COOL-DOWN

STRADDLE REACH *(eight reps each side)*

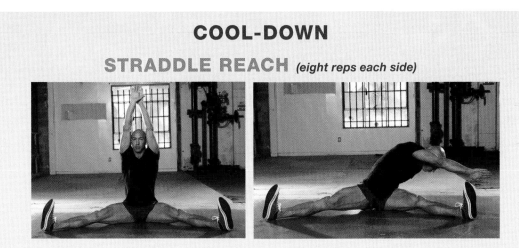

WARM-UP

Jumping Jacks (for sixty seconds)

Then do eight reps of each of these exercises, for two rounds total:

SIDE-LYING LEG LIFTS   ITB LEG LIFTS   BACKSTROKE

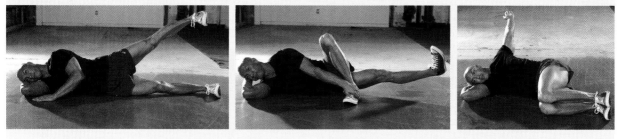

WORKOUT

60/00 WORK-TO-REST INTERVALS.

DOUBLE FUN GLIDE

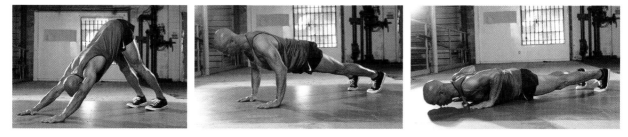

LET ME UPS

TIPS: Your first priority is making yourself perfectly straight by getting your hips up, tightening your abs, and getting your head positioned properly.

Your second priority is going all the way *down* each rep.

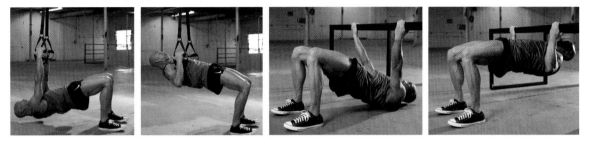

STREAMLINE ROMANIAN DEAD LIFT (WEIGHTED OPTION)

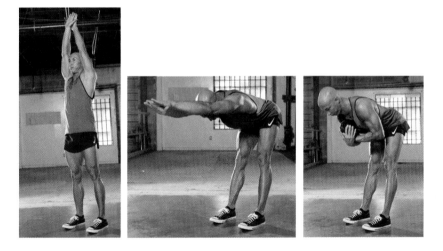

COOL-DOWN
ISOMETRIC PIGEON STRETCH
(8 x 10 seconds on each side)

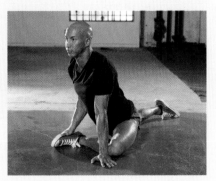

WARM-UP

March in Place (for sixty seconds)

Then do eight reps of each of these exercises, for two rounds total:

HIP CIRCLES   TWIST AND REACH   POINTERS

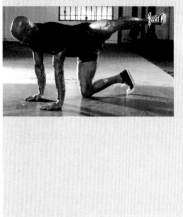
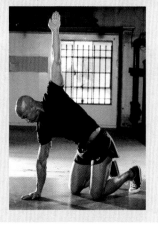
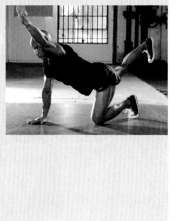

WORKOUT

50/10 WORK-TO-REST INTERVALS.

ARM HAULERS

TIP: Exhale as you swing your arms past your head.

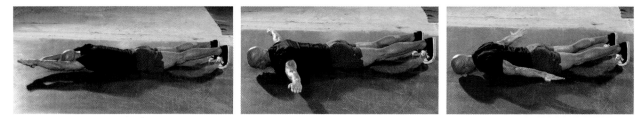

SIDE KICK

TIP: Exhale in each of the Kickout and Side Kick positions.

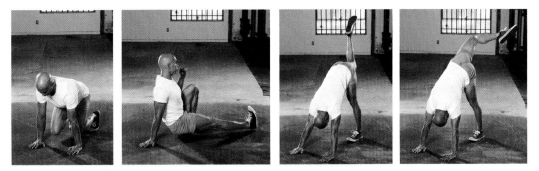

SQUAT TO ROMANIAN DEAD LIFT

TIPS: Sync up your breathing with your other movements. Inhale as you squat down. Exhale as you transition to the bottom of the Romanian Dead Lift.

Inhale as you transition back to the bottom of the T-Arm Squat. Exhale fully as you stand up tall and straight.

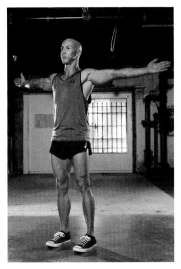

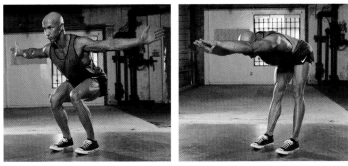

COOL-DOWN

HIP ROLLS *(eight slow reps)*

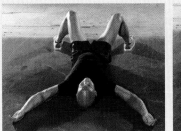
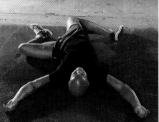
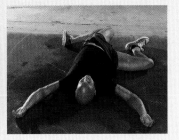

You did it!

As we'd say in Spec Ops, *HOOYA!*—meaning,

"GIVE ME MORE!"

So here's some more: You can repeat cycles 3 and 4 endlessly or head on over to marklauren.com/strongandlean for more 6-week cycles. And here's how you'll continue to make gains:

1. Increasing the reps of each exercise.

2. Increasing the quality of your movements. Controlling every body part and keeping it in its precise, proper place drives progress. Again, perfect performance = perfect physique.

But first, take a week off! Have fun!

And come show us what you've done at marklauren.com/strongandlean.

Just keep locomoting if you can. Go for a couple of long walks and you'll be ready to start cycle 3 the following week!

Stay consistent.

Stay perfect.

ACKNOWLEDGMENTS

We'd both like to thank our editor, Daniela Rapp, for not only helping us realize our vision but making it a joy.

Joshua: I'd like to thank my old Marine buddy Leighton for years ago telling me, "There needs to be a book about bodyweight exercises out there!"

And most of all, I'd like to thank my mother, the strongest woman I've ever met, who unwaveringly championed all my creative efforts.

Mark: Creating these exercise programs has been a team effort. I need to thank Raphael Ruiz and my Master trainers Lea Badenhoop and Christopher Alt for their ongoing support. I also owe the people of Thailand a giant thank-you. My interactions with your culture ignited a curiosity in me that sharply accelerated my learning and allowed me to develop an intense appreciation for all things basic and necessary.